Retterhouse
3/23/06
#36.95

W9-BTD-366

Caring Science as
Sacred Science

Caring Science as Sacred Science

Jean Watson, PhD, RN, HNC, FAAN
Distinguished Professor of Nursing
Murchinson-Scoville Chair in Caring Science
University of Colorado Health Sciences Center
School of Nursing
Denver, Colorado
Jean.Watson@UCHSC.edu
Web Site: www.uchsc.edu/nursing/caring

 F. A. DAVIS COMPANY · Philadelphia

RT
84.5
W366
2005

F. A. Davis Company
1915 Arch Street
Philadelphia, PA 19103
www.fadavis.com

Copyright © 2005 by F. A. Davis Company

Copyright © 2005 by F. A. Davis Company. All rights reserved. This book is protected by copyright. No part of it may be reproduced, stored in a retrieval system, or transmitted in any form or by any means, electronic, mechanical, photocopying, recording, or otherwise, without written permission from the publisher.

Printed in the United States of America

Last digit indicates print number: 10 9 8 7 6 5 4 3 2 1

Acquisitions Editor: Joanne Patzek DaCunha, RN, MSN
Development Editor: Kristin L. Kern
Project Editor: Danielle J. Barsky

As new scientific information becomes available through basic and clinical research, recommended treatments and drug therapies undergo changes. The author(s) and publisher have done everything possible to make this book accurate, up to date, and in accord with accepted standards at the time of publication. The author(s), editors, and publisher are not responsible for errors or omissions or for consequences from application of the book, and make no warranty, expressed or implied, in regard to the contents of the book. Any practice described in this book should be applied by the reader in accordance with professional standards of care used in regard to the unique circumstances that may apply in each situation. The reader is advised always to check product information (package inserts) for changes and new information regarding dose and contraindications before administering any drug. Caution is especially urged when using new or infrequently ordered drugs.

Library of Congress Cataloging-in-Publication Data

Library of Congress Cataloging-in-Publication Data

Watson, Jean, 1940-
    Caring science as sacred science / by Jean Watson.— 1st ed.
        p. ; cm.
    Includes bibliographical references.
    ISBN 0-8036-1169-2 (hardcover : alk. paper)
    1. Nursing—Philosophy.   2. Nursing ethics.   3. Caring.
    [DNLM: 1. Nursing Care.   2. Ethics.   3. Nurse-Patient Relations.
    WY 100 W3395c 2005] I. Title.
    RT84.5.W366 2005
    610.73—dc22

                                                        2004001936

Authorization to photocopy items for internal or personal use, or the internal or personal use of specific clients, is granted by F. A. Davis Company for users registered with the Copyright Clearance Center (CCC) Transactional Reporting Service, provided that the fee of $.10 per copy is paid directly to CCC, 222 Rosewood Drive, Danvers, MA 01923. For those organizations that have been granted a photocopy license by CCC, a separate system of payment has been arranged. The fee code for users of the Transactional Reporting Service is: 8036-1169-2/04 0 + $.10.

The image on the cover is generally referred to as "The Brighton Angel," a statue located on the seafront facing the City of Brighton, Sussex, England. Underneath the statue is the inscription: "In the year 1912 the inhabitants of Brighton and Hove provided a home for the Queen's Nurses and erected this monument in memory of King Edward VII and as a testimony of their enduring loyalty."

Photo by John R. Tuttle. © 2004. Used by permission.

"You know, they often speak of ethics to describe what I do, but what interests me when all is said and done is not ethics, not only ethics, it's the holy, the holiness of the holy

(*i.e.*, saint, las saintete du saint).
Emmanuel Levinas
(in Critchley & Bernasconi, 2002, p. 27)

To all those engaged in caring practices who await discovery of the sacred nature of their work; discovery that they are honored as gifts of humanity, offering divine service to the world. It is through such practices that humanity is sustained across time and space and we are awakened to new realities of Caring in its simple and profound forms of knowing-being-doing as the ultimate manifestation of Infinite Love of healing work in the world. My continual gratitude goes to the students, practitioners, and colleagues around the world as well as to a new generation of children/grandchildren who are doing/being/becoming this model.

My special appreciation and thanks to Jim Irwin, who offered precision and patience with the editing and detail work on this manuscript, helping to bring it to completion, and to Joanne DaCunha at FA Davis for her trust, confidence, continuing support, and patience during the birth of this book.

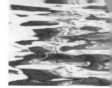

Could the professional deathbed of sorts that we face today in our conventional medical and nursing world be an opportunity for health professionals and scholars to reconsider how we may wish to live our personal/professional lives? How might we wish to carry out our professional/personal calling if we were to pause, to ponder deeper spiritual meanings for the nature of our work and our life purpose. What and how might we approach this time to heal and be healed within and among our professions, with so much unfinished business that has accumulated over the past century?

How might we offer up our heart when we may be disheartened or in fear? As Kierkegaard put it: how do we encounter *"our sickness unto death?"* How do we exist in this in-between existence, where spirit and matter have been torn apart, split asunder, from our identity, our existence, our very Being? Revisiting such foundational issues of Infinity of humanity in relation to our caring and healing may be the difference between life and death of individuals and of professions. Perhaps it is only when we acknowledge how much pain and suffering there is in our broken hearts and broken spirits, our broken world, within and without, that we can return to that which is timeless and can offer comfort, peace, and grace; it can both inspire and inspirit us.

This work is unfinished and a work in progress in that it offers pointers toward another way to view science and caring, especially in relation to human experiences, evolution of humankind, and need for individual and global healing in the world. The work may not need to be read in linear order but according to the reader's interest and mood to grasp the spirit of the message.

Native Americans remind us, because they remember why they are here, that every day we should do an act of power and an act of beauty. By considering a new model of science that embraces caring and healing and the deepest depth of our evolving humanity, I offer an act of power and an act of beauty to this effort. In some ways, this work may serve as an exemplar, or metaphor at least, for the mystical experience that connects us in our remembering for this work.

The intent is to explore, reveal, and mirror back another model of science that honors our deepest human experiences and moral longings; the model seeks to tap into noble truths, uncovering what we already know at some deep level. The concepts and frames of reference point toward a Caring Science, but are not *It*. The context and philosophies represent reminders of what and who we are, helping us to remember the moral spirit-filled dimensions of caring work and caring knowledge.

This work has evolved over the past decade and been made more evident through my own personal journey with caring and healing. Tolle (2003) reminds his readers in his latest book, *Stillness Speaks,* of Sutras, ancient Indian teachings, that are powerful pointers to the truth. Sutras do not engage the thinking mind exclusively but tap into vibrations of inner knowing, connecting with words and ancient truths that cause one to pause, to stop, to be still and ponder the Sutra pointers. It is often considered more important to note what is not explained than what is, in that the words and concepts seek to touch the sacred and a state of consciousness Tolle calls stillness or abiding peace. So, with that caution, and that mindset, this work is to be considered beyond itself and not the thing itself. However, I hope, a new path, another pattern for self, science, and society emerges for the reader, helping to align the holy and profane in a new order of human evolution and wisdom, whereby we can consider Caring Science as a hopeful paradigm for a world and a science that has gone astray and is in crisis.

Jean Watson

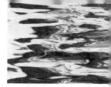

> Seek the wisdom that will untie your knot
> Seek the path
> That demands your whole being.
> Leave that which is not, but appears to be
> Seek that which is, but is not apparent.
> —Rumi, 2001, p. 68.

This work is a call, an invitation, and an evocation for another phase of the journey in science; to embark into a new/old territory that integrates the modern scientific orientation toward the physical material world, with ancient and contemporary wisdoms. These are wisdoms concerning the meaning and destiny of our nonphysical spirit-filled existence, now necessary for preserving the human and our humanity at this crossroads/turning point for humankind. Thus, the call for a worldview, if not a new moral-metaphysical foundation, for our scientific model, even a consideration of a scientific cosmology that simultaneously incorporates the physical with the nonphysical: the empirical with metaphysics and morality, a model that seeks to integrate information with knowledge, knowing with understanding, understanding with wisdom. Indeed, perhaps we need to be reminded once again that the origin of philosophy and science is a search for both knowledge and wisdom that guide our life and our science.

In this work, I have allowed myself to incorporate personal material and *rememberings* to ground some of the ideas and focus. This is my, perhaps, awkward attempt to grasp my own conversation with myself, for my own caring-healing processes, to connect with the deep Being I am meeting and have met *inside, and I am, but am not yet, become/becoming.* So, in some ways, writing about caring and science may not be tolerated in academic circles and scholarly work, but if there was ever a time to converge personal and professional authentic ethical efforts for living/being/doing/becoming scholarly and scientific, it is NOW.

This model of science, which embraces such a distinct orientation, I am calling Caring Science: it is proposed as a model of science that allows us to approach the sacred in our caring-healing work. In and through this book, I am writing what I need to learn as well as what I have learned and continue to learn. It is not only a journey into Science and a new perspective on science, it is also a personal journey into understanding deep caring and how this learning guides others, and me perhaps, into a new, deeper perspective on life and caring-healing work. This name, Caring Science, is neither new to me nor to any of us, once we awaken to our nature and admit our need for inspirations to serve the spirit as well as the body of science and self-alike. Programs and academic departments in Denmark, Finland, Norway, and Sweden (e.g., the works of Kari Martinsen, Norway; and Katie Eriksson, Finland) already use such deep philosophical-ontological-metaphysical language and frameworks of Caring Science to explore caring and its deeper meanings.

Another motivation for my writing this text on Caring Science is because I have the privilege, and indeed the felt honor, of holding the first and only Endowed Chair in Caring Science in the United States and North America, at least to this date: The Murchinson-Scoville Chair in Caring Science, University of Colorado Health Sciences Center, School of Nursing. It is the anonymous and named benefactors who support this direction of my work in the University and the world. Out of this honor, I feel an obligation to try to write about Caring Science at a deeper level that takes us into the emerging future, even though we may not grasp it fully as of yet, but it is on the horizon of an evolving consciousness of humankind.

The exploration toward a Caring Science, to date, has occurred and continues to occur primarily in academic nursing throughout Scandinavia, but it increasingly serves as a foundation for other/all health sciences. However, in North America, Caring Science per se is neither systematically explored nor pursued as a model to better our work and understanding of caring, healing, and health. (The exception is the work of international nursing caring theorists and scholars.)

It is no surprise that Caring Science per se has not been further developed in the Western world because we all know Science is head-brain-cognitively centered; when one enters into a Caring Science model, it opens up a heart-centered connection with our science, ourselves, and all others and our universe.

Ironically, the discipline of nursing during the past three decades has been critiquing and revising its knowledge, assumptions, philosophies, theories, and ethics of caring practice. This scholarly, reflective activity has often been undertaken silently, undetected, outside the halls of mainstream medical science, and even, to some extent, outside the mainstream nursing science foci (Watson, 1995). Nevertheless, some of these works within nursing, as well as changing developments in medicine and science generally, are bearing fruit in introducing new understandings of science, forms of inquiry, methods and practices, reigniting connections between science, art, spirituality, and restoring values, ethics and new relationships between and among heart sciences and humanities and the arts for healing purposes. In addition, there is emergence of new perspectives for exploring contemporary scientific agendas related to complex human caring-healing field phenomena. And many disciplines are now striving to explore models of research for these emerging new healing phenomena, but exploring them from a guiding moral, philosophical foundation.

Caring Science invites and offers another context as well as a conceptual-philosophical-moral and scientific framework that is no longer anomalous with respect to the conventional and nonconventional inquiries and questions being addressed. The rhetorical question may remain: Can we have a science model that is built upon a moral and metaphysical foundation that is made explicit in relation to our humanity and *all our relations*, obligations, one to another? If so, then how are we to Be? Become? Belong in this universe? This work seeks to tap into this rhetorical question.

We nevertheless may protest, argue, and consider (indeed, I even consider it) somewhat of an oxymoron to juxtapose *Caring* with *Science* in that they appear to be incompatible and contradictory, on the face of it, especially viewed from a conventional (natural, biomedical science) lens. As my colleague Dr. Marlaine Smith (1994) put it, we have tension between the dominant scientific paradigms of what has been, in contrast with a vision that is open to what is possible. However, perhaps now the time is right for such paradoxical scientific considerations and integrations, which allow science, morality, metaphysics, art, and spirituality to co-mingle for new reasons. As Sartre suggested, when things are so bad, we long for something else, for what might be, rather than succumb to what is, then we are open to, if not ready for, change.

Science now enters another phase of its journey...it now enters its wisdom phase.

—Brian Swimme, 1996

*Heart, Hand, and Eagle serve as symbols and metaphors for the message in this book. That is, the **Heart** represents deep Love and wisdom, which we seek, long for in our attempt to remember who we are and why we came here, as we pursue our deep knowing and awaken to our true scientific mission: to better our human condition and humanity's evolution. My hope is for offering a return to Love, Belonging, and Caring as the foundation for understanding them as the source for knowledge and wisdom: both empirical as well as metaphysical. The **Hand** reminds us that we literally and figuratively hold another person in our hands, and our hands are also a source of human touch, that touches beyond the body physical and reaches into the* *infinity of the human soul, reminding us of our inter-subjective, transpersonal human-to-human universal connection. The **Eagle** serves as a messenger, a spirit-guide who soars higher than any other bird, closest to spirit world; thus, a reminder that we are spirit-made-whole, and we are connected with both the physical and non-physical nature of our existence and of the existence of an unfolding universe.*

—JW, Sea of Cortez, México, January 29, 2003

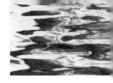

Janet Alexander, RN, MSN, EdD
Associate Professor
Samford University
Ida V. Moffet School of Nursing
Birmingham, Alabama

Barbara Matthews Blanton, RN, MSN
Assistant Clinical Professor
Texas Woman's University
College of Nursing
Dallas, Texas

Jacqueline Fawcett, PhD, FAAN
Professor
University of Massachusetts, Boston
Boston, Massachusetts

Savina Schoenhofer, RN, PhD
Professor
Alcorn State University
Natchez, Mississippi

Susan L. Ward, RN, PhD
Associate Professor
Nebraska Methodist College
Omaha, Nebraska

Table of Contents

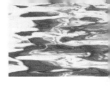

1

Beginnings: Original Text on Caring Science

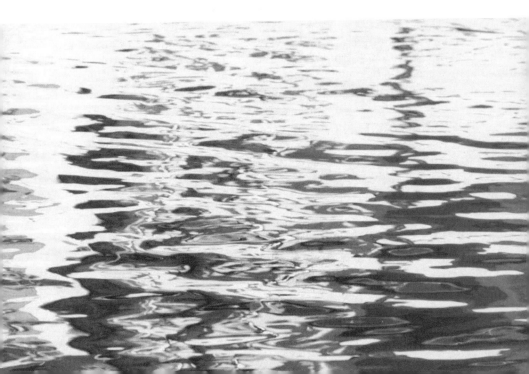

(Watson, J. [1985]. *Nursing: The philosophy and science of caring*. Colorado Associated University Press: Boulder, Colo. [Original work published 1979 by Little Brown: Boston.])

In my first original work on Caring Science, I acknowledged the balance of science and humanities, indicating how the humanities (and arts) address themselves to deeper values of the quality of living and dying, which involve philosophical, ethical, psychosocial, and moral issues. This acknowledgement served to remind us that now it is possible to define an outcome of scientific activity (prolongation of life) without referring to its aesthetic, humanistic aspect (quality of living and dying) (Watson, 1985, p. 3) and certainly not addressing the notion of healing, with living and death/dying. A Science of Caring seeks to integrate and encompass the whole of these phenomena and human experiences.

As noted in the original book on Caring Science:

> there exists the capacity for Science of Caring (to) approach problems from both directions (and maybe today, all directions) . . . combining science with humanities. The Science of Caring cannot remain detached from or indifferent from human emotions—pain, joy, suffering, fear, and anger. At the same time, as its name indicates, the Science of Caring is guided by scientific knowledge, methods, and predictions (Watson, 1985, p. 5, author's parenthesis).

Within the context of an attempt to articulate the core processes of Caring, I identified 10 *Carative Factors* that comprised a tentative foundation for the Science of Caring. This was originally posited as a framework for nursing, which now extends to encompass all health and healing practitioners and professions, at least as a guiding philosophical-ethical-practice model, if not a model for further theory and knowledge development (Watson, 1985, pp. 9–10).

THE ORIGINAL TEN CARATIVE FACTORS

1. The formation of a humanistic-altruistic system of values;

2. The instillation of faith-hope;

3. The cultivation of sensitivity to one's self and to others;

4. The development of a helping-trusting relationship;

5. The promotion and acceptance of the expression of positive and negative feelings;

6. The systematic use of the scientific problem-solving method for decision making (later modified to soften the harsh language of linear process, allowing for creativity, openness with caring process, open to all ways of knowing);

7. The promotion of interpersonal teaching-learning (later refined to read as transpersonal teaching-learning);

8. The provision for a supportive, protective, and/or corrective mental, physical, sociocultural, and spiritual environment;

9. Assistance with the gratification of human needs;

10. Allowance for existential-phenomenological dimensions.

These factors were referred to as the *"core"* for professional practice, which are timeless and enduring, transcending new knowledge, skills, technology, specialty and subspecialty practices, which are referred to as *"trim"* in that (nursing or health-healing) profession cannot be defined and guided philosophically and ethically by its trim alone, as that is always changing.

The changing nature of the Carative Factors will be taken up in a later chapter, indicating their evolution to incorporate a more explicit relationship between Caring and Love, moving toward using the language of **"Caritas,"** closely related to the original term **Carative** but conveying a deep form of transpersonal caring and love to come into play as part of a caring-healing perspective guiding Caring Science (see Appendix 4 and Watson website, **www.uchsc.edu/nursing/caring**).

It is when we include caring and love in our science, we discover our caring-healing professions and disciplines are much more than a detached scientific endeavor, but a life-giving and life-receiving endeavor for humanity.

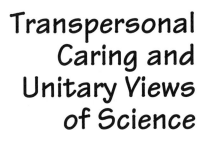

Transpersonal
Caring and
Unitary Views
of Science

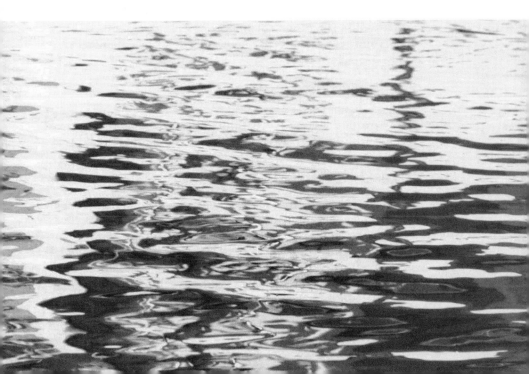

Transpersonal Caring is one extant caring theory (Watson, 1979, 1985, 1988, 1995, 1999a,b), among others, that has emerged as a guide to practice, education, and research for nursing and related fields. Transpersonal Caring is located within a Caring Science framework. The next section provides an overview of some of the basic ingredients of transpersonal caring theory that are related to Caring Science model (Watson & Smith, 2002, p. 458).

TENETS OF TRANSPERSONAL CARING

❊ The transpersonal caring field resides within a unitary field of consciousness and energy that transcend time, space, and physicality (unity of mind/body/spirit/nature/universe);

❊ A transpersonal caring relationship connotes a spirit-to-spirit unitary connection within a caring moment, honoring the embodied spirit of both practitioner and patient, within a unitary field of consciousness;

❊ A transpersonal caring relationship transcends the ego level of both practitioner and patient, creating a caring field with new possibilities for how to be in the moment. "The process goes beyond itself, and becomes part of the life history of each person, as well as part of the larger, deeper complex pattern of life" (Watson, 1985, p. 59);

❊ The practitioner's authentic intentionality and consciousness of caring has a higher frequency of energy than non-caring consciousness, opening up connections to the universal field of consciousness and greater access to one's inner healer;

❊ Transpersonal caring is communicated via the practitioner's energetic patterns of consciousness, intentionality, and authentic presence in a caring relationship;

❊ Caring-healing modalities are often non-invasive, non-intrusive, natural-human, energetic environmental field modalities;

❊ Transpersonal caring promotes self-knowledge, self-control, and self-healing patterns and possibilities;

❊ Advanced transpersonal caring modalities draw upon multiple ways of knowing and being; they encompass ethical and relational caring, along with those intentional consciousness modalities that are energetic in nature, e.g., form, color, light, sound, touch, visual, olfactory, etc., that honor wholeness, healing, comfort, balance, harmony, and well-being.

Caring Science Evolution: Connections Between Tenets of Transpersonal Caring Theory and Science of Unitary Human Beings

The following unifying statements have been identified to make explicit relationships between Transpersonal Caring and Roger's original Science of Unitary Human Beings (Watson & Smith, 2002, pp. 458–459):

❈ The intention of transpersonal caring expands in open, resonating, concentric circles from self to other to Planet Earth to universe. It includes caring consciousness, a heart/mindfulness, while participating knowingly in human-environment field patterning;

❈ The authentic presence, consciousness, and intentionality in a caring moment manifest caring field patterning;

❈ The presence and caring consciousness potentiate change in the field by co-creating human-environment patterning from lower frequencies to higher frequencies (i.e., caring consciousness carries higher energy frequencies than non-caring consciousness);

❈ Transpersonal caring resides within a field of caring consciousness and energy that transcends time, space, and physicality and is one with the universal field of consciousness (spirit)—the infinity.

Transpersonal Caring and Unitary Science

Some of the shared notions between these two frameworks Transpersonal Caring and Science of Unitary Human Beings co-mingle for a Caring Science Unitary model. These trans-theoretical dimensions are outlined in Table 2-1 (Watson & Smith, 2002, p. 459):

Caring and Health as Evolving Consciousness

In addition to the trans-theoretical discourse between Transpersonal Caring Science and Roger's Science of Unitary Human Being discussed above, recent work by Newman (2002) [whose theory evolved from Roger's Unitary Science (1970)] explores specific trans-theoretical connections and commonalities between her works on *Health as Expanding Consciousness and Caring*. She pursues dialectic between caring and knowing, like Gadow (1990), when she acknowledges her notion of "pattern recognition" as "knowing," which can therefore be

Table 2-1

Trans-Theoretical Dimensions of Transpersonal Caring and Unitary Science

TRANSPERSONAL CARING (WATSON, 1988, 1999)	UNITARY SCIENCE (ROGERS, 1970, 1994)
• Transpersonal—transcends time, space, physicality; grounded in the "eternal now"—caring moment; • Universal field of Consciousness—connects with infinity; • Consciousness is energy—caring consciousness manifests high-frequency energy waves; • Body = light, energy, (body resides in universal field of cosmic consciousness; • Mutuality of Caring relationship—transpersonal process.	• Pan dimensionality—a nonlinear domain without spatial or temporal attributes; • Infinity—unitary-transformative worldview; • Resonancy—Principle of continuous change from lower to higher frequency energy wave patterns; • Body—manifestation of energy field; • Integrality—mutual human-environment field process.

Adapted from Watson & Smith, 2002, p. 459. Reprinted by permission.

viewed as a form of *Caring*. The relationship between *Health as Expanding Consciousness* (Newman, 1994) and *Caring Consciousness* (Watson, 1999b) converge.

Newman (2002) identified some overlapping aspects between caring and knowing congruent with both her work and mine (Watson, 1988, 1999, 2000, Website www.uchsc.edu/nursing/caring). In the following key points, I have extracted and integrated key points from Newman (2002, pp. 9–10) and my earlier work as well as current thinking. I, likewise, have transposed the term *Caring* for *Nursing* in the Newman citation, to indicate the universality of Caring, which is emerging among and across other caring-healing professions, as well as making the ideas congruent with Caring Science context.

❋ Caring is about relation and meaning;

❋ Caring is an integrating (perhaps transforming) force for health care (and healing);

❋ Caring is transcending itself in a framework of expanding consciousness;

* Caring, a form of knowing, can be transformed into a more inclusive caring as a higher level of consciousness;

* There is an explicit connection between Caring/Caritas and Love (Watson, 1999, 2002);

* The highest level of Consciousness is Love;

* Expanding Consciousness of Caring evolves toward Cosmic Love as universal life force energy of the universe.

Within this evolving framework: "The dialectic of caring and knowing unfolds in expanding consciousness, which is revealed in greater Caring. The highest level of consciousness is Love" (Newman, 2002, p. 9). These comparisons highlight some of the congruence between the moral-metaphysical positions of Levinas and Logstrup, to be discussed in more depth, and Caring Science with its focus on Transpersonal Unitary dimensions espoused by Nursing Theorists. Upon reflection one can see the relationship between these emerging metaphysical worldviews for Caring Science and emerging philosophies and theories in this area.

3

Extant Caring Theories as Metaphysical, Meta-Ethical, Meta-Narrative to Guide Caring Science

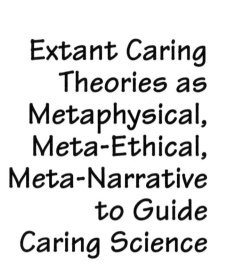

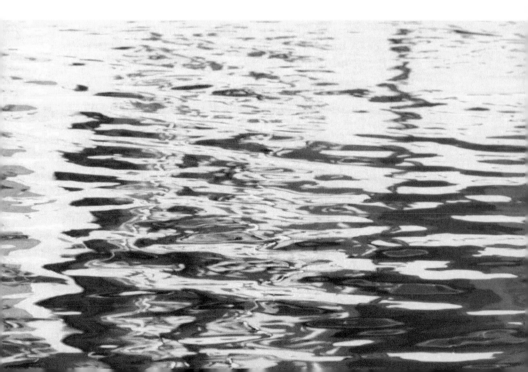

Extant theories of caring offer various views on caring that may be considered Grand Theories. Grand Theories are global, abstract context for phenomena that frame disciplinary knowledge. Grand Theories transcend specific events and seek to provide universal explanations that reflect ethical-philosophical foundation and values for the entire field of study (Reed, Shearer, & Nicoll, 2003).

What is distinctive is that in each case, across the theories, there is an underlying metaphysical-ontological foundation that locates Caring Science in a moral-philosophical-ethical context to guide science and practices alike. For example, a classic synthesis of the caring theories by Smith (1999) explored caring at the ontological-ethical level. She was able to clarify how caring knowledge resides within a holistic context honoring the unitary of human-in-relation. Smith's work uncovered five constitutive meanings of caring from a wide range of caring theories (from the nursing literature). These findings explicate the ethical, metaphysical, and relational ontology of Caring, which contribute to a Caring Science orientation. These findings are consistent with the philosophical ethical ground that European philosophers Levinas (1969) and Logstrup (1997) offer as a contemporary perspective to re-think science and Caring Science as a specific case for Science. These philosophical-metaphysical and empirical findings of caring from the theoretical literature include the following (Smith, 1999, pp. 22–25):

❋ Caring is a Way of Manifesting Intentions: (e.g., Person-centered intention; Preserving dignity and humanity; Committed to alleviating vulnerability; Giving attention and concern; Reverence for person and human life; Love and co-presence; Authenticity and availability; Being with; Compassion, Regard; Intentional presence; Knowing, Acknowledging, Affirming, Celebrating Other);

❋ Caring is a Way of Appreciating Pattern: (e.g., Placing value on the Other as lovable, worthy of being loved; Cherishing the wholeness of the human being; Assuming the subjectivity of Other as valid and whole; Acknowledging the emerging pattern of Other without trying to change it; Seeing the Other as perfect in the moment; Unfolding possibilities for becoming; Yearning for a deeper understanding and appreciation of the natural healing resources, life force, pattern and paradox; Sensitivity to pattern manifestation that gives identity to each unique person; Transcending judgment; Seeing beyond fragmentation to existence of wholeness).

❋ Caring is a Way of Attuning to Dynamic Flow: (e.g., Attuned to subtleties in the moment; Sensitivity to self and Other; Connected; Belonging and Interconnected; Living in context of relational; Detecting the person's Being and feeling the condition; Synchronization and organismic integration; Action of Love; Energetic resonance; Pattern or vibration of consciousness becoming attuned with Other).

❋ Caring is a Way of Experiencing the Infinite: (e.g., Transcends physical and material world, bound in time and space; Expanded sense of self: transcendent qualities; Highest form of knowing; Unfolding divine Love; Ontological mystery; Spiritual union—transcending self, time, and space; Spirit of both present, expands the limits of openness; Caring moment relations between past-present and imagined future).

❋ Caring is a Way of Inviting Creative Emergence: (e.g., Holding hopeful orientation; Growing in capacity to express caring; Transforming mutual process; Caring action—growth of spiritual life within; Calling to deeper life-birthing spiritual life in each person; Expanding human capacities; Facilitating creative emergence).

EMPIRICAL UNDERSTANDINGS OF CARING

The theoretical and empirical work of Swanson (1991, 1999) has made an important contribution to Caring Science knowledge and understanding. Her phenomenological investigations of women experiencing perinatal loss lead to her development of an empirically derived middle-range theory of caring that was later empirically validated (Swanson, 1991). Through her extensive work, she defined caring as "a nurturing way of relating to a valued other towards whom one feels a personal sense of commitment and responsibility" (Swanson, 1991, p. 42). In her theoretical framework, she defined five processes through which caring is manifested:

❋ *Knowing*—striving to understand an event as it has meaning in the life of Other;

❋ *Being with*—being emotionally present and available;

❋ *Doing for*—doing for Other what they would do for themselves if at all possible;

❋ *Enabling*—facilitating the Other's passage through life events and transitions by providing information, validation, and support; and

❀ *Maintaining belief*—sustaining faith in the capacity of the Other to get through events or transitions and face a future with meaning.

In addition to her empirical and theoretical work on caring, Swanson also conducted a classic meta-analysis of the state of caring science knowledge as extracted from nursing research literature (Swanson, 1999). This analysis of 130 empirical nursing research studies offers further evidence as to the importance of caring knowledge and the consequences of caring and non-caring for both patients and nurses (in these instances). For example, some of the empirical findings with respect to both positive and negative outcomes of both caring and non-caring are in the following two tables (see Tables 3-1 and 3-2).

While the summary of these studies was based upon nursing research on caring, the implications are there for all health professionals. The importance of both structure and processes whereby caring occurs at the deeply human level for both patients and practitioners seems to be critical with respect to outcomes for both sides.

Table 3-1

Empirical Outcomes of Caring Research for Patients (Based upon Meta-analysis of 130 empirical studies)

CONSEQUENCES OF CARING	CONSEQUENCES OF NON-CARING
SUMMARY OF RESEARCH OUTCOMES OF *CARING* FOR *PATIENTS*	SUMMARY OF RESEARCH OUTCOMES OF *NON-CARING* FOR *PATIENTS*
• Emotional-spiritual well-being; dignity, self-control, personhood; • Physical enhanced healing; lives saved, safety, more energy, less costs, more comfort, less loss; • Trust relationships, decrease in alienation, closer family relations.	• Humiliated, frightened, out of control, despair, helplessness, alienation, vulnerability, lingering bad memories; • Decreased healing

Swanson, 1999.

Table 3-2

Empirical Outcomes of Caring Research for Nurses (Based upon Meta-analysis of 130 empirical studies)

CONSEQUENCES OF CARING	CONSEQUENCES OF NON-CARING
SUMMARY RESEARCH OUTCOMES OF *CARING* FOR *NURSES*	SUMMARY RESEARCH OUTCOMES OF *NON-CARING* FOR *NURSES*
• Emotional-spiritual sense of accomplishment, satisfaction, purpose, gratitude; • Preserved integrity, fulfillment, wholeness, self-esteem; • Living own philosophy; • Respect for life, death; • Reflective; • Love of nursing, increased knowledge	• Hardened • Oblivious • Depressed • Frightened • Worn down, etc.

Swanson, 1999.

Bio-nature Continuum of Caring Relationships

Other manifestations of the critical nature of the human-to-human relationship in caring-healing practices are revealed in some of the classic research in Iceland by Halldorsdottir (1991). Halldorsdottir's work on nurse-patient relationships revealed five types of relationships that classify a continuum from uncaring to caring. They include the following:

❋ Type 1: Biocidic or life-destroying (toxic, leading to anger, despair, and decreased well-being);

❋ Type 2: Biostatic or life-restraining—cold or treated as a nuisance;

❋ Type 3: Biopassive—life-neutral—apathetic or detached;

❋ Type 4: Bioactive—life-sustaining (classic nurse-patient relationship as kind, concerned, and benevolent);

❋ Type 5: Biogenic—life-giving, mutuality and interconnectedness, openness to Love, giving and receiving in the moment.

This research has critical moral and practical implications, in that the biocidic relationship is one in which the patient is actually harmed by the practitioner, through manipulation, coercion, abuse, humiliation, or other forms of physical, mental, emotional, or spiritual violence. It "involves the transfer of negative energy or darkness to the other" (Halldorsdottir, 1991, p. 39) whereas the Biogenic—life giving mode of Caring parallels the "Caring Moment" (Watson, 1988, 1999) whereby the caring consciousness (Biogenic response) energetically emanates a quality of positive, if not loving, energy that potentiates healing. There is a spirit-to-spirit, soul-to-soul connection between the two people in a caring (biogenic) moment. Both share a new field that goes beyond either person and that has a field of its own that is greater than the moment itself. The process goes beyond itself, yet arises from this moment of connection, becoming part of the life history of each person as well as part of some larger, deeper, complex pattern of life (Watson, 1999a, p. 59). These views open us to notions of infinity and mystery of relationships and the impact of one person's humanity upon another.

This way of considering our humanity and influence in Others' life and world, for better or for worse, is congruent with French philosopher Levinas' (1969) notion of moral, primordial notions of how we approach life and Other. In early writings on Caring, I put it this way: "each person has to question his or her own essence and moral behavior toward others, because if people are dehumanized at a basic level, for example a human care level, that dehumanizing process is not capable of reflecting humanity back on itself" (Watson, 1988, 1999, p. 50). Indeed, this is perhaps what Levinas refers to as *turning our face away* from our humanity, with dangers of *totalizing* another and humanity itself, becoming faceless, anonymous, and indifferent to our humanness. So, in our day-to-day relationships, as well as in the caring moments of professional practice, we pause to comprehend the profound implications this theoretical and philosophical work has for our scientific work and our world.

By expanding our discourse on science, on caring knowledge, theories, ethics, and practice phenomena, a trans-theoretical, trans-disciplinary development unfolds as a new philosophical-ethical foundation. New possibilities can and do exist for the emerging caring-healing scientific field and the wider arena of human health sciences (Watson & Smith, 2002) in that we can better attain the mandate to *at least do no harm*. Our consciousness, intentionality, and very presence can and do make a difference in a person's life, for better or for worse. Again, Logstrup (1997) reminded us: *we literally hold another person in our hands.* This *moral orientation for caring is beyond science and epistemology but holds approaches to Caring Science in its hands.*

At their most basic level, healing and health care involve a human caring, relational moral process as the essence of their professional practice. They exist by virtue of an ethical-moral ideal and commitment to provide both a scientific and humane, human service to others, with the hopes of helping another achieve a sense of wholeness, dignity, and *right relation* (Quinn, personal communication, 1991) in a way that transcends any medical treatment, disease, or diagnosis.

Anyone engaged in caring healing practices plays a prominent role within the relationship itself, in helping to preserve humanity, integrity, and human dignity within their care practices as well as the systems that deliver care. An intentional focus on caring and healing practices helps to sustain caring in the midst of threats, biological or otherwise (Watson, 1988, 1999a).

The literature on caring from the field of nursing is the most prominent source of work on the epistemic and philosophical-theoretical nature of caring. In addition to the findings above, further literature posited caring as a "human model of being" (Roach, 1987). Caring has been noted as a basic way of "being-in-the-world and creating both self and world" (Benner & Wrubel, 1989, p. 398).

Recent Disciplinary Directions Affirming Caring in Nursing

(Excerpt adapted from Watson, J. [2002]. *Assessing and measuring caring in nursing and health science.* NY: Springer, pp. 13–14. Reprinted with permission.)

In addition to the above developments within nursing science, some other major events attest to the centrality of caring as part of nursing's focus, which increasingly has relevance to other health sciences, including for example the following evidence:

❀ Academic structures and departments in Scandinavian countries named "Caring Science";

❀ Two international journals with a focus on Caring: *Scandinavian Journal of Caring Science* and *International Journal of Human Caring*;

❀ International Professional Organization: International Association of Human Caring (IAHC) celebrated its 25th year (2003);

* "Caring Science": *The Science of Caring* Research Publications (University of California, San Francisco, School of Nursing), over 15 years old;

* Key recommendations for caring as core concept for nursing— National Reports: American Academy of Nursing (AAN) Wingspread Conference;

* National League for Nursing (NLN) curriculum standards;

* Special devoted monographs, conferences, journal issues on Caring;

* American Nurses Association (ANA) revised definition—Social policy statement with inclusion of caring and caring relationship as core aspect of nursing practice (1995).

This accumulation of converging developments helps to resolve the dissonance about caring and its place within the discipline of nursing; moreover, this momentum now serves as a foundation and context for emerging Caring Science, which has relevance for all health sciences.

However, it is clear today that nursing is not alone in identifying care issues and outcomes; indeed, other disciplines now are recognizing and incorporating caring into their frameworks. For example:

* Caring-healing modalities and therapeutics and their effects are emerging among a range of diverse practitioners and health-basic scientists;

* Relationship-centered care/caring as a major initiative among health care reform systems and individuals (Fetzer Institute Project of Relationship-centered Care; www.fetzer.org);

* Feminist studies and women's health;

* Ethics, philosophy, and educational fold;

* Emergence of Caring Science as an academic discipline in its own right (e.g., Eriksson, K & Lindstrm, U. [1999]. *A theory of science for caring science*. Hoitotiede. 11[6], pp. 358–364).

Thus, from the nursing field, and throughout these emerging trends in the growing field, Caring has increasing relevance and interest to the care of people and our world. In addition, in considering Caring as a moral as well as epistemic endeavor, Caring has been framed consistently as a relational ontology, with ethical spiritual overtones, which take precedence over epistemology, or at least offer directions to better inform Caring epistemology, research, and practice models. This view is consistent with Levinas' (1969) philosophical position, except he made it clear that Ethics was the first philosophy and came before ontology for itself alone. That is, Belonging is the relational and ethical starting point, which comes before our being and knowing, and invites us into an ethical moral response as part of our actions.

Assumptions Related to Human Caring

Some basic assumptions related to Human Caring have been defined as follows (Watson, 1988, 1999a, pp. 32–33, with slight modification):

❊ Caring and Love are the most universal, the most tremendous and the most mysterious of cosmic forces; they comprise the primal and universal psychic energy;

❊ Often these needs are overlooked; or we know people need each other in loving and caring ways, but often we do not behave well toward each other. If our humanness is to survive, however, we need to become more caring and loving to nourish our humanity and evolve as a (world) civilization and live together;

❊ (Our) . . . ability to sustain (our) caring ideal and ideology in practice will affect the human development of civilization and determine (health profession's) contribution to society;

❊ As a beginning we have to impose our own will to care and love upon our own behavior and not on others. We have to treat ourselves with gentleness, loving kindness, equanimity, and dignity before we can respect and care for others with gentleness, kindness, equanimity, and dignity;

❊ Society is in a critical situation today in sustaining human caring ideals and a caring ideology in practice . . . . At the same time there has been a proliferation of curing and radical treatment cure techniques often without regards to costs (or human/humanity considerations);

❊ Health professions' social, moral, and scientific contributions to humankind and society lay their commitment to human caring ideals (and ethics) in theory, practice and research.

In summary, the basic metaphysical-moral orientation and assumptions related to Human Caring and its relationship to caring knowledge and practices are congruent with the philosophical foundation of Levinas, (1969). His notion of *Ethics of Face* and Infinity, as discussed throughout this text, as well as Logstrup's (1997) ethical demand are both related to the moral fact that we both literally and metaphorically *hold another person's life in our hands.*

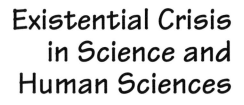

Existential Crisis
in Science and
Human Sciences

Continuing Journey
Toward Caring Science

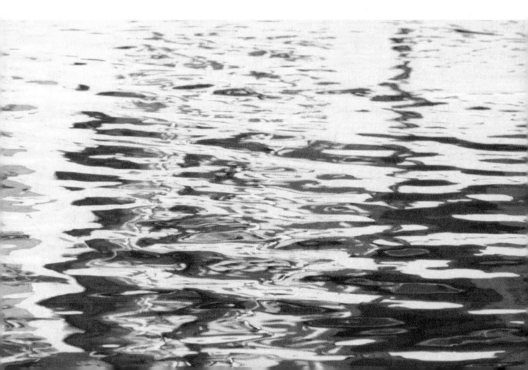

Even the so-called Human Sciences, with their various attempts to incorporate new assumptions for science, have had their existential crises in the past half-century. There have been the rise and fall of Grand Theory to guide history and philosophy of science to an overthrow of all Grand Theory and any attempts to construct a systematic view of the nature of human and society, in spite of major sociological-historical intellectual movements. Ironically, with this crisis, it has led back to Grand Theory for new reasons, as this chapter explores.

Thus, there have been various waves of philosophical scientific thinking in the human science discourse and directions. For example, Laslett in Skinner (1994) pointed out that historically there was an effort toward the abandonment of the

> study of grand philosophical systems of the past, with their unsatisfactory mixture of descriptive and evaluative elements, in order to get on with the truly scientific and purportedly value-neutral task of constructing what came to be called 'empirical theories' of social behavior and development. The effect of all of this was to make it appear that two millennia of philosophizing about the social world had suddenly come to an end (Laslett, 1956, p. 4 in Skinner, 1994, my italics).

This momentum against Grand Theory partially contributed to the purely empirical science fixation, which discarded the substantive moral, metaphysical, and even epistemological issues of the day. Within the history and philosophy of science generally, the positivist account of what counted as knowledge and explanation became dominant (i.e., see Hempel, 1965, pp. 245–295 in Skinner, 1994, p. 4). The influence of Karl Popper and his disciples exercised an enormous influence toward a generally "rationalist" stance, requiring any experiment to be subjected to attempts to "falsify it, thus separating anything factual from anything metaphysical or normative." Only then, in Popper's view, according to Skinner, were human science and social science phenomena on the road of the straight and narrow path to becoming genuine sciences (Skinner, 1994, p. 4).

Nursing science in particular has followed this scientific-theoretical momentum and the enticement with the rise and fall of Grand Theory, parallel with social-philosophical movements in Europe and the Western World of science. For example, with the overturn of Grand Theory, there likewise has been a recent tendency toward abandonment of nursing theories and the subsequent moral-metaphysical underpinnings they provide for research and the very phenomena of human caring and healing nursing seeks to study. However, the changing turn toward a moral and philosophical foundation for nursing supports the current rise in Grand Theory again, to offer a meta-narrative for a discipline.

Historically, however, the ironic rise of postmodern thinking and the deconstructive movement in literary, historical, and philosophical-scientific circles in Europe, and later around the world, contributed to, first, the paradoxical abandonment, and, more recently, the return to Grand Theory to guide philosophies of science and research. As Skinner (1994, p. 7) pointed out in his book *The Return of Grand Theory in the Human Sciences,* "times have certainly changed" and once again new philosophies are being practiced, revived, and are flourishing in a variety of forms. Witness the widespread influence of Michel Foucault, Hans-Georg Gadamer, Jacques Derrida, Jürgen Habermas, and others, including the whole range of previously neglected arguments from Feminist studies and the Women's Movement in general.

One of the dominant themes in all these developments/transformations in the history and philosophy of science has been the dominant discourse, even widespread reaction, against the assumption that the "natural sciences offer an adequate or even a relevant model for the practice of social (human) disciplines" (Skinner, 1994, p. 6, my parenthesis). Basically this critique has reminded us that the positivist contention that all successful explanations must conform to the same deductive model of physical-natural sciences is misconceived. The claim of course is that the attempt to recover and interpret meaning (related to human experience) and social actions must include, and even take the form of, the point of view of the persons themselves (Skinner, 1994). Even the best attempts to address human science phenomena were challenged by these thinkers, challenging the routines and disciplines of society and science, to resist and deconstruct, if not "destroy, the so-called scientific movement, in the name of (saving) our own humanity" (Skinner, 1994, p. 10, my parenthesis).

Such strong sentiments, ironically, led to a new grand narrative about knowledge and how to approach questions of epistemology; thus injecting or reasserting anti-theory as a paradoxical Grand Theory view. This was the result of the postmodern turn by the various philosophers and historians of science according to Skinner (1994).

The inadvertent result ironically has now resulted in this movement toward reintroduction of Grand Theory. This turn has occurred more by default than by purpose, or as a result of some of the unexpected consequences of the deconstructivist movement. What seemed to occur in the beginning was a new grand narrative evolution that rejected any overriding theory or worldview; however, in the process of deconstruction of the negative side-effects of classical science, the new postmodern movement resulted in a stripping away of the underlying values, moral foundation, and metaphysical ground for science and theory alike. Once ideas are deconstructed to their core, theory and science alike are into nihilism and moral abyss (Watson, 1999a). Thus, then, the ironic rise of Grand Theory to offer a necessary meta-view, a meta-narrative of philosophical-ethical foundation for a discipline; otherwise it loses its values, its moral map, its meaning and purpose.

Therefore, a return to an ethical, philosophical foundation for our science helps us relocate our professional knowledge and ourselves in practices that are congruent with our experiences and our larger world. This takes us to an ironic turn back to Grand Theory as meta-narrative for a metaphysical-ethical starting point. This turn allows for a Caring Science that can accommodate some of the existential crises and angst of the postmodern deconstructivist consequences of the Human Science attempts as well as consequences of the classic assumptions for conventional science. Both rigid conformity to classic assumptions as well as total deconstruction of all approaches toward theory and science are equally faulty. Caring Science mediates the two extremes by trying to unify the best of a moral-metaphysical foundation with pluralistic epistemologies and methodologies. This perspective views a cosmos that is at the same time both unitary and multiple, both One and Many: within this cosmos are many spiritual centers of consciousness: one is physical, which houses the spirit; another, a pantheistic world in which spirit is both immanent and transcendent, leading to the ultimate unspeakable mystery. Such a world is *alive; sacramental* (Reason, 1993).

Reason (1993) makes an explicit relationship between metaphysics and science by acknowledging the profound contradictions to the secularized experience, knowledge, and action of Western society and its science. He points out that if we are to live our lives as high-quality inquiry, we need to consider inquiry as sacred.

He makes a case for sacred experience and sacred science. From this perspective, he advocates for "reverential thinking" for the appreciative and sensitive mind, reverence for life, appearing as a natural acknowledgement of the miracle and beauty of life itself (Reason, 1993).

Reason goes on to suggest that personal experiences and study of the epistemological crises of our world can lead to scientific inquiry that is grounded in immediate experience of the presence of the world and contained within a wider cosmology; so an essentially mystic/spiritual worldview underpins both Reason's and Fox's view about quality in human inquiry (Reason, 1993; Fox, 1988).

Such a view toward the sacred in science reminds us of the fact that the human person is "a fundamental spiritual reality with a distinct presence in the world" (Heron, 1992, p. 52).

The notion of a living, sacred cosmos, within Reason's view, can inform our notions of inquiry so we can develop a new kind of sacred science. Thus, such a science that restores the metaphysical integrates "a critical, self-reflexive consciousness with a deep experience of the sacred, and would thus make a major contribution to what Maslow (1971) referred to as the 'further reaches' of human nature" (Reason, 1993).

5

Working Assumptions for Caring Science

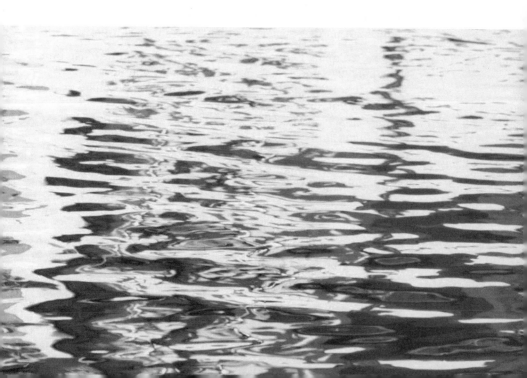

Thus, a Caring Science that seeks to unify, rather than separate, is based upon a different set of assumptions:

* An Ontological assumption of oneness, wholeness, unity, relatedness, and connectedness;

* An epistemological assumption that there are multiple ways of knowing, not only the physical sense data, but through tapping into our deep humanity our caring-healing relationships with self, Other, Nature, one's inner belief, accessing the infinity of life force of the universe, opening to something greater than oneself;

* Diversity of knowing assumes all, and various forms of evidence can be included, e.g., commonly identified areas such as empirics, but subjective, aesthetic, noetic, poetic, personal, intuitive, ethical, mystical, and spiritual knowing. (It can be noted that in some ways some of these are already included in normative science and theory when notions such as "elegance," "beauty," "simplicity," and "parsimony" are used when choosing alternative theoretical-scientific explanations around a phenomenon [Harman, 1990, 1991; Fawcett, Watson, Neuman, & Hinton-Walker, 2001]).

* A Caring Science model makes these diverse perspectives explicitly and directly;

* Moral-metaphysical integration with science evokes spirit; this orientation is not only possible but also necessary for our science, humanity, society-civilization, and world-planet.

* Finally, a Caring Science emergence, founded on new assumptions makes explicit an expanding unitary, energetic worldview with a relational human caring ethic and ontology as its starting point; once energy is incorporated into a unitary caring science perspective we can affirm a deep relational ethic, spirit, and science that transcends all duality. As this thinking evolves, we open to the infinite, which invites the sacred to return to our professions and science (Watson & Smith, 2002, p. 459).

The following additional considerations are ways to frame a Caring Science model (Watson & Smith, 2002, p. 456):

* Developing knowledge of caring cannot be assumed; it is a philosophical-ethical-epistemic endeavor that requires ongoing

explication and development of theory, philosophy, and ethics, along with diverse methods of caring inquiry that inform caring-healing practices (and knowledge);

❋ Caring Science is grounded in a relational ontology of unity within the universe, which in turn informs the epistemology, methodology, pedagogy, and praxis of caring;

❋ Caring Science embraces epistemological pluralism, seeking the underdeveloped intersection between arts and humanities and clinical sciences, which accommodates diverse ways of knowing, being-becoming, evolving; it encompasses ethical, intuitive, personal, empirical, aesthetic, and even spiritual/metaphysical ways of knowing and being.

Caring Science inquiry encompasses methodological pluralism, whereby the method flows from the phenomenon of concern, not the other way around; the diverse forms of inquiry seek to unify ontological, philosophical, ethical, and theoretical views, while incorporating empirics and technology (Watson & Smith, 2002, p. 456, author's parenthesis).

6

Metaphysics and Science

Can There Be a Re/Union?

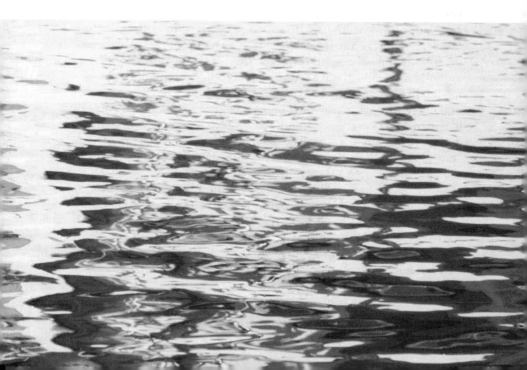

... the much desired union of science and metaphysics (would) lead the positive sciences, properly called, to become conscious of their true scope, often far greater than they imagine.

Henri Bergson (In Harman, 1991, p. 6)

In spite of some of the latest writings of Ken Wilber (2001) (http://wilber.shambhala.com/html/misc/habermas/index.cfm/cfm/xid,58 37/yid,5049275), who has a view on post-metaphysical spirituality and post-metaphysical thinking with respect to science, the efforts in this work seek to make a case for a moral, metaphysical foundation for Caring Science.

Wilber (2001) acknowledges on his Website that he categorically rejects metaphysical approaches, in that he agrees that metaphysics is concerned with understanding the (higher) world, whereas science is concerned with facts and evidence (Website, p. 3). He, of course, puts his "faith" in rationality, rejecting any non-evidential views of "faith." However, at the same time, he is "allowing for postmodern levels of consciousness, as phenomenological occasions, ultimately revealed as Spirit's potential for transcendence and known directly by a good broad science" (Website, p. 8).

There is almost a paradox in his model, because of his broad/deep science views for a reconstructed science. For example, he rejects anything on ontological levels of faith for defining reality; nevertheless, he has developed an integral epistemological model that allows all the evidence to be included, embracing spirit and subjectivity. In that sense, his views are congruent with the direction that I am trying to point toward for a Caring Science; however, I would not call this view post-metaphysical. Indeed, in Caring Science, I too subscribe to "evidence" and reconstructing science as he proposes, as well as including subjective data that flow from the inner world of spirit, indi- vidually and collectively. Without going into the complexities of Wilber's model, I think there is both congruence and difference with his views and evolving notions for Caring Science. For example, he differentiates between "narrow science" (only real is sensorimotor, rational, theoretic) and "broad science" or deep science, which can only be seen with the "inward eye" (Website, p. 5). Wilber suggests that all forms of "good science," e.g., narrow, broad/deep, or reconstructed science conforms or follows three common features: e.g., exemplars/paradigm; empiricism (experiential grounded); and potential for refutation. Each of these strands is followed in all forms of "science": sensory, mental, and spiri- tual science (Wilber, 2001, p. 5).

Where I think I differ from Wilber is in his rejection of metaphys- ical grounding for "science"; I differ in his rejection of faith at ontological level; indeed, to revert to Kierkegaard, at some point, in sorting out our reality, we must "take a leap of faith" for our moral grounding to sustain caring and life itself. This view, it seems to me, is especially relevant when trying to point toward Caring Science specifically.

Toward these differences, Harman (1991) actually made a case for the reunion of science in metaphysics, in that metaphysics has different meanings. I am choosing to adhere to both forms of meanings in making a case for reunion of metaphysics and science for a Caring Science model. Taylor (1974) likewise made a case historically in the need for metaphysics. It seems to me that metaphysics is what offers the basic ontological, moral meaning about humanity and life/death itself, all phenomena of critical importance to caring and healing work.

However, with Wilber's scheme for knowledge, as we see later in the formal figure, his framework of integrality offers a congruent, conceptual model for knowledge development and caring-healing phenomena; that is, it accommodates both matter and spirit; phenomenological-empirical; individual and collective; objective and subjective/experiential. All of these, in Wilber's model, can indeed be explored with empirical data, just of a different kind of what counts as evidence, allowing for phenomenological sciences: different levels/states of consciousness (gross, subtle, and causal) (Wilber, 2001, p. 5) that allows research on spiritual practices, experiential insights, mediations, spontaneous healing, non-local consciousness, etc. The view here is consistent with the fact that data are needed for Caring Science; it is just that with a Caring Science model I wish to make explicit a metaphysical foundation. I do so, not to make a case for an irrational belief system, which Wilber rejects, but rather to make explicit a moral foundation and worldview that embraces Caring and Healing, also within a reconstructivist model of science in its own right. Thus, Caring Science as being pointed toward here, both overlaps with and differs from Wilber's view on a post-metaphysical science. I am not alone in this view of need for metaphysics.

A CASE FOR METAPHYSICS

Richard Taylor is known for his treatise on metaphysics, where he reminds us that there are many things one can do without, but one of the things one cannot do without, at least "not without deep suffering and the diminishing of our human nature, is the love of at least a few . . . others" (Taylor, 1974, p. 40–41). Another need he identified that one cannot do without, or that "cannot be destroyed or left unmet without great damage . . . is the love for nature and the feeling of our place within it" (Taylor, 1974, p. 41).

The other such need he identifies for human survival is the need for metaphysics herself. He points out she "does not promise the usual rewards that a scientific knowledge of the world so stingily withholds . . . . Metaphysics in fact promises no knowledge of anything . . . then what is her reward? What makes it worth seeking at all?" (Taylor, 1974, p. 42) He goes on to exclaim that the need for metaphysics endures to save us from the numberless substitutes that are constantly invented. However, her path is not easy, and no certain treasure lies at the end, and people will choose substitutes for metaphysics. "Yet it is only metaphysics that, while preserving one in the deepest ignorance . . . will nevertheless give that which alone is worth holding to . . . . For metaphysics promises wisdom, a wisdom sometimes inseparable from ignorance, but whose glow is nevertheless genuine . . ." (Taylor, 1974, pp. 43–44).

Without going into a whole treatise on the history and philosophy of science, it is important to offer a general context for the discussion of science and metaphysics. It is necessary to be reminded why they have become so incompatible in modern thinking and science and how Caring Science seeks to overcome these seemingly incompatible restrictions and separations.

Willis Harman's (1990, 1991) earlier work attempted to make a case for the *reunion* of science and metaphysics, reminding us that during the early period (Royal Society, founded in 1660) science and metaphysics were so intertwined as to be two aspects of a single endeavor. Early founders and members of the Royal Society, such as Robert Boyle and Christopher Wren, were also steeped in the esoteric and metaphysical traditions of the day. It also helps to be reminded "the term 'metaphysics' has two very different meanings. The first definition refers to metaphysics as a branch of philosophy; comprising both ontology and epistemology; the second to the study of the transcendent or supersensible reality" (Harman, 1990, 1991, p. 6). Caring Science embraces metaphysics in the broader meaning comprising both ontology and epistemology, which likewise honors the transcendent within it as a branch of philosophy. And more specifically, within Levinas' framework, philosophy is first principle for knowing/knowledge/ science.

To consider the notion of Caring Science and its reconciliation with metaphysical and moral considerations, it is necessary to consider how what has come to be the classical assumptions of modern science keep us tied to a separatist ontology, limited epistemological horizons, and restrictions on our forms our inquiry that shape our knowledge, our ways of knowing, and our entire worldview. For example, the underlying dominating, classic assumptions of modern science are/have been:

- The ontological assumption of separateness; an epistemological assumption that all knowledge is based on physical sense data that are measurable;
- Hence, the methodological assumption to study a phenomenon required it to be reduced to its most elemental parts, smaller and smaller units, separated from the whole. (Harman, 1990, 1991).

These three classical assumptions, framed as *Objectivism, Positivism, and Reductionism,* have shaped not only modern science but also our very view of reality and what is true and valued. It is no wonder that the metaphysical starting point for our philosophies and theories of science and reality are disconnected from our human experiences and lived world. Within such a view of reality and science, there is no room for phenomena and happenings that require another starting point: acknowledgement of connections versus separations.

The original scientific ontological and epistemological assumptions of separateness and control of physical reality have had lasting and lingering implications, whereby we continue to posit and pursue methods that detach and separate observer and observed; human from environment (nature); mind from body/matter; parts from a whole; science from source, and so on. That is not to say that the part cannot and should not be studied. It is just recognizing it belongs to a whole, and in reality the whole is already in the part. Nevertheless, the ingrained mental notion of separation and its limited ways of knowing have been absolutely fundamental to our mindset and our worldview and remain so, although this is beginning to change. As a historian, philosopher, and educator, Whitehead reminded us the modern mind had a vehement and passionate interest in the relation of general principles to "irreducible and stubborn facts" (Whitehead, 1925, p. 3) and how this state of mind impacted upon spiritual forces in our life and kept these so-called stubborn facts separate from anything spirit-filled.

This separatist view has likewise separated the academic and professional disciplines from each other, including nursing and other health sciences from medicine, and caring science from medical science, specifically. However, this assumption has now reached a point of humility in recognizing we are not, and cannot remain, in separate isolation; now it is true, for moral-ethical reasons as well as scientific-economic survival reasons.

Within the field of medical science, of caring and healing research and practices, there are increasing accounts of phenomena that do not conform to the classic scientific assumptions of separateness, objectivism, and reductionism; for example, the evolving work in psycho-neuro-immunology, distant healing, prayer, love research, spontaneous-natural healings, cardio-energetics, energy nursing/medicine, healing relationships, self-healing approaches, not to mention the exploding field now more commonly referred to as complementary-alternative practices.

These new phenomena have been identified within the multiple contexts of, for example, non-local consciousness, Unitary-Transformative Frameworks, Unitary Science, New Paradigm Research, Wholeness Science, Extended Science, Holographic Paradigm, and so forth. (For more depth in these frameworks, see some of the works of Bohm, 1980, Dossey, 1991, Harman, 1990, 1991, Newman, 1992, Reason, 1988, Rogers, 1970, 1994, Wilber, 1982). Each of these perspectives acknowledges multiple ways of knowing, being, and doing research and science that connect human and nature/universe, honoring an infinite inner wisdom of the mind-body-spirit-universe lattice network, connecting us with the infinity of the universe. Such emerging frameworks are open, curious, exploratory, and honoring, even surrendering to, ineffable explanations, acknowledging the mysteries and miracles happening in our midst. All of these contemporary emerging mindsets for science and natural life processes defy the classic, dominating assumptions that have been adopted for modern scientific thinking.

However, in spite of the classic mindset for modern science and its metaphysical assumptions, it is important to acknowledge that different views of science specify a point of view, from which the field is conceptualized, the assumptions that are inherent in that claim, and the basis upon which knowledge claims are accepted. Differing views of science also reflect the differences between a biomedical-oriented science and a social, human caring-oriented science (Watson, 1995, p. 66). As differing views of knowledge are unveiled and insights evolve about our science models and assumptions, we become more aware of explicit approaches toward a human-caring science that often conflict metaphysically, philosophically, and morally with conventional classic science assumptions and principles: For example, (Watson, 1995):

❀ The clinical, mechanistic-medicalized concept of person conflicts with the concept of unitary person in relation to others and the infinity of the universe;

❀ The study of human beings reducible to body parts or sum of the parts; without recognizing/acknowledging notions like spirit, energy, subjectivity, consciousness, and the irreducibility of mind-body-spirit;

❄ The static model of science conflicts with continuously evolving self-organizing fields of change;

❄ Objectifying phenomena as detached and separated from the whole is in conflict with whole person relational perspectives.

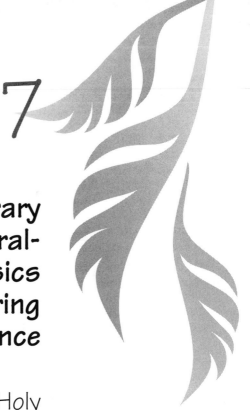

7

A Contemporary Case for Moral-Metaphysics Ground for Caring Science

Approaching the Holy and the Sacred

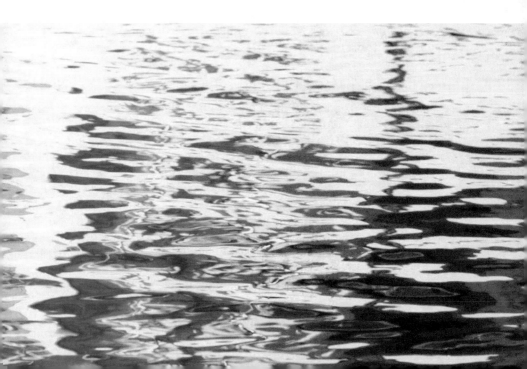

Still another such need, strangely, is the need for metaphysics herself . . . .
What am I: What is death—and more puzzling still, what is birth? A beginning? An ending? . . . , does it matter?

Richard Taylor, 1974

There is such a close connection between French Philosopher Emmanuel Levinas' philosophy in particular, and as discussed later, Danish Philosopher Knud Logstrup. The next section goes into more depth of Levinas' work and its more explicit connection with notions of Caring Science. Later a section on Logstrup integrates the two philosophies for a Caring Science lens. It is these very foundational dimensions of life itself, that perhaps we have paid too little attention to, which now require our attention here for new reasons.

Critchley reports that, at Levinas' funeral, Derrida recalled a conversation with Levinas in Paris. "Levinas said, 'You know, they often speak of ethics to describe what I do, but what interests me when all is said and done is not ethics, not only ethics, it's the holy, the holiness of the holy'" (*le saint, le sainteté du saint* [Critchley & Bernasconi, 2002, p. 27]). In this direction of considering this thinking and this work on Caring Science, we are led to another, deeper perspective of life that is related to notions of love and peace, which will be taken up later. But for purposes here, we are reminded by Levinas, Logstrup, and caring and unitary theorists that there is a unity and holiness to life, a mystery that is unfathomable and that Levinas captured by claiming that the true source of wonder, with which philosophy supposedly begins, is not "to be found by staring into the starry heavens, but by *looking into another's eyes, for here is a more palpable infinity that can never exhaust one's curiosity . . .* " (Critchley & Bernasconi, 2002, p. 27, author's italics).

EMMANUEL LEVINAS: HIS INFLUENCE FOR CARING SCIENCE

Levinas was reported to be fond of saying the entirety of his philosophy could be "summarized in the simple words, '*Après vous, Monsieur/(Madame)*'" (Critchley & Bernasconi, 2002, p. 27), in that these expressions and behaviors capture the most everyday acts of civility, hospitality, kindness, consideration, politeness, and, yes, I might add, *Caring*. Such a basic perspective brings to mind clinical situations in which we may pause in the midst of all the clinical dramas and ethical dilemmas and maybe ask the simple question: What would be the kind thing to do in this situation? What would be the kindest thing we could do? Such reflection posed by my physician colleague in the United Kingdom, Dr. Sarah Eagger (2001), totally changes our clinical mindsets of professional ego controls and invites basic human considerations to prevail. I have to think that this is what Levinas had in mind, if he or we were to manifest this deeply human moral thinking in the midst of our often chaotic professional practice.

In this framework the ego is put into question, the professional-disciplinary boundaries are transcended. The point of location for Being is outside our personal and professional egos, and ourselves; it becomes *Otherness*, what Levinas called *"exteriority,"* that cannot be reduced to the cognitive, ego enterprise (Critchley & Bernasconi, 2002, p. 15). This way of thinking becomes so basic, it may be thought of as banal (Critchley & Bernasconi, 2002), but becomes the most fundamental essence of our existence and a moral and metaphysical map and guide for sustaining caring, healing, and even our humanity at a time of its threat of survival in the world. As a foundation for this deeply moral-metaphysical understanding, Levinas does not necessarily claim to be providing us with "new knowledge or fresh discoveries, but rather with what Wittgenstein calls *reminders* of what we already know but continually pass over in our day-to-day life" (Critchley & Bernasconi, 2002, p. 7).

When we consider shifting our basic moral professional and disciplinary foundation for caring healing science and practice from detached preoccupation with external, objective *Evidence* toward *Values-Based Practice*, and when we consider/reconsider Values we reach deep into our roots of humanity and help to restore the moral light that guides authentic caring inquiry and actions. To consider this deep level of moral foundation that plumbs the depth of our humanity, which Levinas presents, it becomes an invitation to restore the heart of our professions and our healing.

As Dr. Sarah Eagger (personal communication, 2001—International Association of Human Caring conference presentation, University of Stirling, Scotland) put it:

> A profession without values becomes heartless;
> a profession that loses it heart is soul-less;
> any profession that becomes heartless and
> soul-less becomes worthless.

By considering the depths of Caring and Healing as both science and practice as informed by contemporary work of Levinas, Logstrup, and the extant caring field, we bring values back as the moral-metaphysical foundation and starting point, lest we become worthless professions. (See Appendix A for Table with an overview of these major philosophers/philosophies.)

By restoring this moral values–guided foundation, we renew our energy and clarify our *raison d'etre for Being, and are indeed reminded of why we are here: To Love, Serve, and Remember* (Astin, 1991).

The writings of Emmanuel Levinas, the contemporary French philosopher (1906–1995), invite all health professions interested in caring and healing into this new/old metaphysical space for our science and practices. Levinas' work has received widespread appeal in scientific and philosophical circles in recent years. As Critchley reports, quoting Jean-Luc Marion, Professor of Philosophy at the Sorbonne (Paris), "If one defines a great philosopher as someone without whom philosophy would not have been what it is, then in France there are two great philosophers of the twentieth century: Bergson and Levinas" (Critchley & Bernasconi, 2002, p. 2). It is also generally agreed that Levinas was largely responsible for the introduction of Husserl and Heidegger in France. He completed his doctoral thesis on Husserl, in which, as Critchley reports, Levinas jokingly suggested that he (Levinas) introduced Jean-Paul Sartre to phenomenology.

As I understand one of the core aspects of Levinas' work, he critiqued and differed from Heidegger in ways that upset mainstream thinking in philosophy. His departure from Heidegger, with respect to metaphysics and moral-ethics of *Belonging (as relational-ethical ontology) coming before Ontology of Being, just for itself,* has become one of the fundamental starting points for his work. His work provides powerful, rich, and complex descriptions of a whole range of phenomena. However, as Critchley notes: "Levinas' one big thing is expressed in his thesis that ethics is first philosophy, where ethics is understood as a relation of infinite responsibility to the other person" (Critchley & Bernasconi, 2002, p. 6). These other powerful and rich phenomena that are closely related to this text and Caring Science include, for example:

❉ Levinas' concept of *Ethics of Face;*

❉ The deep-lived sensibility of an embodied exposure to the Other, which is worthy of deep subjective experience;

❉ His notion of "psychism"—relational responsibility or responsivity to the Other; this *psychism*, what other traditions may call the "soul," is what is calling me/you to respond.

In turn, this "soul" resides in mystery; it is connected with the Infinity of the Universe, of the Universal field of Infinite Love "by looking into another's eyes, for here is a more palpable infinity that can never exhaust . . . " (Critchley & Bernasconi, 2002, p. 27).

Many and diverse disciplines are now pondering, integrating, and inquiring into this complex and engaging moral-metaphysical disciplinary foundation of Levinas' thinking. All of these provocative depths of inquiry and the *call to Other* (through the infinity of soul, witnessed and lived through Face-to-Face being) have drawn a great deal of interest and influence by scholars across such diverse fields as, for example, feminist theory and research, post-colonial cultural theory, theology, Jewish studies, aesthetics, art theory, social and political theory, international relations theory, pedagogy, psychotherapy and counseling, and nursing and medical practice (Critchley & Bernasconi, 2002, p. 5). Indeed, Levinas has become almost an obligatory reference point across most contemporary disciplines (Critchley & Bernasconi, 2002).

Caring Science is no exception. Indeed, Levinas' thinking provides both a moral and metaphysical foundation for helping to clarify why Caring Science is different from conventional science and offers a different starting point.

In drawing upon Levinas in *Totality and Infinity* (1969) and the emphasis Critchley and Bernasconi (2002) brings to our understanding of Levinas in his *Cambridge Companion to Levinas*, our comprehension of philosophy for science at a deep level of understanding can be explored. We can find an understanding that transcends the dominant classic assumptions of a separatist ontology of Being as the starting point for our science and practices. We also can find an understanding that transcends some of the rejection of Grand Theory when it comes to rejecting a common moral-metaphysical ground for caring-healing knowledge and practices and relocate values in our return to Grand Theory as a moral map, and first principle, for our science.

In his philosophy, Levinas makes a case for *Being which presupposes an ethical relation with the other human being,* that *Being to whom I speak and to whom I am obliged before being comprehended.* In this view, fundamental ontology for a starting point for science related to caring-healing in this instance becomes explicitly and fundamentally ethical and relational (therefore, the separation model and classic scientific assumptions, or the rejection of Grand Theory in Human science movement, cannot hold for fundamentally human relational-ethical reasons). It is this very ethical relation that is "*metaphysical, and survives any declaration of the end of metaphysics* (or Grand Theory)" (Critchley & Bernasconi, 2002, p. 10, my italics) in contemporary philosophy of science and, I might add, in any science that attempts to embrace human caring and healing phenomena.

Levinas acknowledged ethics is not reducible to epistemology: "ethics is otherwise than knowledge" (Levinas, in Critchley & Bernasconi 2002, p. 11). Without the astute attention to an ethic and ontology of relation, of Ethics and Philosophy as First Principle, as Levinas puts it, the worst might happen in our science, our relations, our society, our civilization; that is, "the failure to acknowledge the humanity of the other" (Critchley & Bernasconi, 2002, p. 13).

"Such . . . is what took place in the Shoah and in countless other disasters of this century, where the other person becomes a faceless face in the crowd, someone whom the passer-by simply passes by, someone whose life or death is for me a matter of indifference" (Critchley & Bernasconi, 2002, p. 13).

Facing ourself and our humanity . . .
Is a moral act
And comes before clinical knowledge;
. . . the value laden human condition . . .
vulnerability, pain, suffering and discomfort,
are value-laden phenomena;
they are moral realities
(Nortvedt, 2000, p. 2)

ETHICS OF FACE

I am blinded by the light of your face . . . Rumi, 2001, p. 48.
The reflection of your face turns the water into a golden shimmer and softens even the fire into a tender glow, when I see your face, the Moon and the few floating stars around it lose their glory.

Rumi, 2001, p. 14.

The ethical danger in a separatist model of science is it being void of any meta-ethical stance, when the scientific-theoretical work involves caring for others when they are most vulnerable. A separatist model reduces other to separate other, to object other, to It. A separatist model of science separates mind from body, eliminates any sense of spirit; such an orientation to science separates human from environment, from each other, from cosmos, which it seeks to control and manipulate as separate from one's own experience, one's own Being. Without a metaphysical foundation, the conventional separatist model sets up a situation where another human being can be reduced to the moral status of an object. When one is in an object status, the ones with more information, power, and control can begin to justify doing something to other as *faceless object* that they would never do to fully functional Other. When one has a *face-to-face* acknowledgement through the very human contact that connects, we are united through a shared humanity that extends to infinity of humankind, to the Infinity of the Universe.

In Levinas' ethical-philosophical structure, the ethical relation of one to another is not outside the experience as a spectator, but this ethical relation is the opposite of totalizing and is described in terms of infinity. Infinity refers to thinking the fact that I, from the first, "*thinks more than it thinks*" (Critchley & Bernasconi, 2002, p. 14).

It seems that Levinas' view opens us to the artistic sensitivity to being human, to facing our own and another's humanity, and that its objective is a healing act in and of itself. It takes place in any caring moment (Watson, 1988, 1999) where there is authentic human encounter and engagement, spirit-to-spirit, soul-to-soul, and face-to-face. This thesis grounds the artistry of being human, in unitary connection with Other and all of life, and from a Levinasian view is the foundation of Caring Science at its primordial core.

What Levinas refers to as looking into the *face of Other*, as in *facing our humanity through the face*, we touch and connect with the Infinity and beauty of the human soul; one person reflects and mirrors this infinity back to the other. This mystery is that which unites and cannot be turned away from.

When you show your face even the stones begin to dance with joy.
Rumi, 2001, p. 14.

The failure to acknowledge the humanity of the Other, to *turn our face away* from Other as faceless object, Levinas referred to as a *totalizing* of the Other. This turning away can be an act of cruelty, an inhumane act that diminishes our shared humanity; that is, totalizing or objectifying Other is through conceiving of the relation to the Other from some imagined point that would be outside of it and where I can turn myself into a theoretical spectator . . . on the world of which I/we am/are really part, and in which I/we am/are an agent.

For Levinas, meaning and Infinity are contained already in the Face of the Other, and all recourse to words takes place already within the primordial Face-to-Face language (Levinas, 1969, p. 206; referenced in Nortvedt, 2000, p.6). Thus, for Levinas the encounter with Other . . . with the Face is the primary event of Being, both metaphorically and literally, . . . and this basic Ethic becomes *first philosophy*, the metaphysical-moral ground of humanity, and comes before Ontology.

It is in this sense that Belonging to Other, connecting us with the Infinity of the universe, differs from Heidegger's notion of Being for itself alone. So, in this framework, *Belonging* comes *before Being*, as pre-existent and primordial. With Levinasian philosophy and ethic, to comprehend our situation is not to define it as much as to find ourselves in an affective disposition toward it. This reality, before the fact, becomes a basic truth of our humanity and a means to both face and sustain our humanity.

One of Levinas' main claims, which makes it one of the most

contemporary views for us to consider and is Beyond Heidegger, is that Levinas acknowledges that the ontological movement in philosophy fails to appreciate the ethical foundation of Being-in-the-World. Thus, in Levinas' *Ethics as First Principle* and first philosophy indicates that "in openness to the human face, being addressed by its vulnerability, by its 'nudity', moral responsibility sets the scene" (Levinas, 1969, p. xx). The ethical event of encountering the Other breaks with Ontology and Being for itself alone. Thus, Levinas makes a case for metaphysics before ontology in that it sets up the ethics for any philosophical position; indeed ethics becomes First principle.

To be more specific and perhaps metaphorical as well as realistic:

> A look, a glance, a gaze, a touch, a voice which invites and welcomes. A Face which connects with the Infinity of humanity itself, rather than a turning away, is beyond clinical . . . it is entering into humanity itself and the infinity of the universe (Levinas, in Nortvedt, 2000, p. 12).

In Levinas' view, the ethics and artistry of Face become a moral act and come before clinical knowledge (Nortvedt, 2000). But, in this approach, knowledge is not shattered, it is initiated. But the values, the artistry/ethic of being human, come before knowledge and shape and inform the knowledge we use.

As Parker Palmer noted: "It is here, in our modes of knowing, that we shape souls by the shape of our knowledge" (1987, p. 19). This wisdom and insight of Parker Palmer, renowned educator and trans-former of educative minds, has more meaning than otherwise imagined when placed within the framework of Emmanuel Levinas and his ethics of face and view of ethics as being otherwise than knowledge per se. However, this integration of the metaphysical-ethical with the science model does not mean we cannot be scientific with respect to caring-healing and health phenomena, while still honoring the stark reality that ethics and metaphysics of our Being-in-relation come before our science and continue to uncover our faulty assumptions of classical science, which is objectivism, positivism, reductionism, and separatism. Levinas overcomes such faulty assumptions by addressing a view of Infinity and the human soul to which we belong before we are ever separate individuals. The next section explores these dimensions of Levinas.

LEVINAS' VIEW OF INFINITY—SOUL

The concept of Infinity in Levinasian philosophy is honoring the spirituality of "Other," in that therein lies the concept of Infinity. By honoring Other, we comprehend and reveal the Other as mystery, mystical. When we gaze into the eyes of another, we gaze into Infinity. This is a fundamental ethical stance. And to turn away from another, to refuse to face another, that is, to face our own humanity, to turn away from another, is to turn away from Infinity of life itself. And this, therefore, leads to an appropriation or a totalizing, an objectifying of Other and ultimately, in turn, an objectifying of self. In this way of thinking, the union with Other recognizes the Infinity of Subjectivity and the depth of Other. This, in turn, allows us to experience our own mystery and infinity, as one person's level of humanity and infinity of soul reflect back onto us.

This notion of Infinity and Soul grounds Caring, not just with tending to another. But a spiritual orientation with self is founded in Infinity and mystery of the soul of the Other, as reflected/revealed through the Face, and in facing Other in this deep metaphysical way. In this moral manner of relation, both subjects in the caring moment (Watson, 1988, 1999) share their vulnerabilities, founded in the depth of the Other's humanity; in surrendering to the mutuality of Other and self and our relation with the infinity of the universe. The value-laden human condition, which involves caring, is not merely a "matter of providing a service unaffected, as if the patient is only an object of concern, and not a subject, a person living his life in front of us . . . is also opening up toward the human other" (Nortvedt, 2000, p. 4). Thus, the other, as well as the nature of the phenomena, touches a practitioner or scientist in this field morally; this is ethically and epistemologically significant. Whether one deliberately chooses to acknowledge this or not, one is encountering the human destiny of the other, and this has an evident appeal to moral value (Nortvedt, 2000).

In this sense, Caring Science is ethical because it is linked with human well-being, wholeness, and healing in the highest and finest sense of their meaning. Such moral-ethical concerns have deep significance and consequences in that protection, suffering, and relief are related to how another is touched by such significant ethical phenomena of another's living experiences. In Levinas' language, there is hospitality, a welcoming of the vulnerable other, related to receptivity and openness to the other.

Finally, in explicating this view, we acknowledge that ethics, art, and artistry of Being-Becoming are in no way antithetical to knowledge. Rather, ethics, art, and artistry precede knowledge in the sense of being prior to it and welcome it. The encounter with Other is the signification; the Other is an event of particularity: his or her vulnerability, hurt, pain, grief, and so on. Awakened human values, human compassion, caring responses allow us to Face humanity itself and become what Nortvedt (2000) calls the Primordial core of clinical knowledge and care practices, even if we are not aware or awake to what it is we are being/doing in the caring-healing relational moment. It is in this foundational way of remembering that through turning and facing the Other, we are facing and turning toward, and sustaining, not only caring, but humanity itself.

> *Always,*
> *The most important hour*
> *is the Present.*
> *Always,*
> *The most important person*
> *Is the one you are Facing.*
> *Always,*
> *The most important act*
> *Is Love.*
> Meister Eckehart
> *(Courtesy of Ruth Ahrens, Germany, personal communication,*
> *February, 2003)*

8

The Ethical Demand

Knud Logstrup— Holding Other in Our Hands

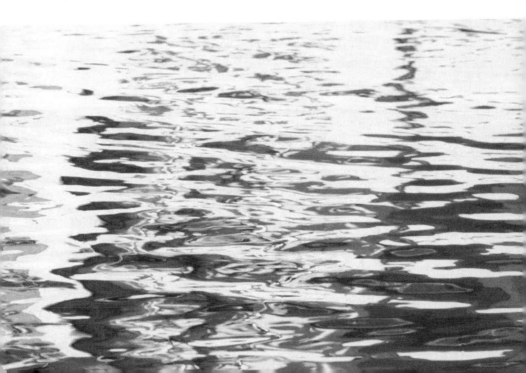

This next section builds upon and extends Levinas' notion of *Face* and its implications for Caring Science. It moves into the metaphorical and literal philosophical framework of Danish Philosopher Knud Logstrup (1997), who reminds us that we *hold another in our hands*; thus we have an ethical demand to attend to this reality in our life and work, especially within a context of Caring Science.

Logstrup's work has become more prominent since his death in 1981; however, his philosophy has gained increasingly more importance in recent discourses in philosophy, ethics, and theology alike. One of the most evocative aspects of his thinking, which is congruent with Levinas' insights, is removing the subject as the sovereign controller of the universe and freedom from engagement with life. His work takes on a very personal touch, using metaphors and images that captivate the imagination. For example, he indicates that within the conventional European philosophies, "the 'I' has been seen as separated from both its life and its world and made into the sovereign subject of the activity of giving form to everything. This isolation of the subject from life and the world is also its isolation from other subjects" (Logstrup, 1997, p. xx). Thus, the I-Thou relationship is reduced to an I-It relationship. He specifically deviated from Heidegger and, like Levinas, makes a strong case for an alternative view.

Logstrup's alternative perspective raises the reality that life itself has already been created with forms and laws of its own. "Life has been given to us and it is a precondition of any cultural ordering that the basic expression of life is both to receive and give. Life, thus, is necessarily interpersonal (if not transpersonal), and involves that basic trust which informs all communication" (Logstrup, 1997, p. xxi). This alternative insight points out that our lives presuppose facts not of our own making and are prior to reason, emotion, and will, facts that invite a spiritual interpretation. This view is grounded in immediate experience of the presence of the world, yet contained within a wider cosmology, a sacred cosmos, both unitary and multiple, both One and Many (Reason, 1993).

Logstrup reminds us that the moral content of life is as it is actually lived; he makes a distinction between sovereign expressions of life and more ego expressions of life, which he refers to as recurrent or obsessive expressions of life. Examples of the latter are attitudes, expressions, and actions expressive of jealousy, hatred, envy, self-righteousness, betrayal, control, greed, etc. These ego-focused expressions related to self as Subject for itself alone contain negative emotional qualities and hold negative energy. However, *the true sovereign expressions of life are expressive actions and attitudes such as trust, honesty, fidelity, solidarity, love, gratitude, caring, forgiveness, authenticity, and so on.*

These emotional expressions, referred to by Logstrup as *sovereign,* intersect with some of the latest thinking regarding consciousness and energetic thoughts; for example, Zukav (1990) viewed the relationship between consciousness, energy, and light as part of our thought systems. Emotions portrayed as currents of energy with different frequencies also are consistent with Rogers' Science of Unitary Human Beings (1970). That is, emotions we think of as negative, such as hatred, envy, disdain, and fear, have a lower frequency and less energy than emotions we think of as positive, in Logstrup's term: sovereign. Examples are those emotions and expressions such as affection, joy, love, compassion (and caring) (Watson, 1999b, pp. 111–112).

The poet Anne Waldman put it this way: "Words are energy. Physical and psychic heat and force" (Waldman, 2001, p. 178).

The so-called sovereign expressions in Logstrup's philosophy are those with higher frequency of energy in contemporary energetic field consciousness frameworks. Again, as we continue to evolve in our human field consciousness toward more caring, loving thoughts, we move toward what Teilhard de Chardin referred to as the Omega Point, a higher level of God-Creator consciousness. This level of evolving moves humanity toward more awareness and honoring of our divinity. This is consistent with not only Chardin's view but also Whitehead's philosophical perspective, in that they envisioned humanity as co-participating in our evolving, unfolding universe, and reminds us that the highest level of consciousness is Love.

Back to Logstrup's view, with respect to these human expressions: he reminds us we are not the cause/controller of such sovereign expressions of our life. "They are not mine/our achievement, but through them I/we can achieve what will be of genuine help to others" (Logstrup, 1997, p. xxv). They become sovereign, because in them *"my life has taken me over before I have taken my life over"* (p. xxv).

These perspectives are not confined to a *system* of moral philosophy, but a *living* philosophy of engagement, honoring the gift of life, which has been given to us, before the fact of our control over it. Indeed, the sovereignty of such basic human expressions of Belonging-Being-Becoming more human and humane becomes Logstrup's *ethical demand,* for it is only through others that we receive the content for our experiences, from which they arise. And at the same time the situation and our engagement transform the situation. It is because only in and through them are we open, active, engaged, spontaneous, authentic. And through this realization, we also realize we are neither the cause nor the controller of these sovereign expressions in our life. They are not my achievement, but given to me/us as possibilities that the I cannot make use of for its own individual purposes alone, but through which it can more fully realize itself/its humanity, becoming more connected, engaged, alive, open, and spontaneous.

In this way of reframing our views of humanity, Logstrup's ethic shifts the emphasis from the ethical demand itself to those sovereign expressions of life, which are the fulfillment of the demands. He makes it clear that while we cannot always will to perform such non-ego expressions and actions, which are these sovereign expressions in our life, we likewise cannot prevent them from finding expression in our life, as the very nature of our humanity. They are not at our disposal to create; they are given to us as the gift of being alive. The demand then is that we should let those sovereign expressions of life that we know to be good be sovereign in our own lives. This is a radical demand and in many ways unfulfillable while, at the same time, an ethical ideal and guide for caring-healing professionals.

These sovereign expressions and the ethical demand of Logstrup's views intersect with transpersonal caring theory and the living out of caring in a *caring moment*, in relation with other; the ethical demand in this instance is to respond from those sovereign expressions in our life that present themselves in any *caring occasion and can manifest as a caring moment, which in turn becomes transpersonal—it is both immanent and transcendent* (Watson, 1988, 1999). It is important to note that "the demand" is not the other person in the situation, per se, but the fact that "the demand" makes itself and does so impersonally because our life is not of our own making. The demand requires of me that I act for the sake of this particular other human being or set of human beings. This response to such a demand is beyond the universality and generality of moral rules, but presents itself in concrete situations in the moment. I am doing what is required and appropriate.

Thus, the key part of understanding Logstrup is to remember at some deep level that *our life is not of our own making. We did not create it!* Something is given prior to and as a precondition for all that we may think and do (Logstrup, 1997, p. xxix). This perspective moves us very close to a philosophical foundation for honoring the sacred gift of life as beyond us and our making and control, but rather something that we yield, submit, and surrender to in its most concrete, honoring, holy sense.

Logstrup's work has a close working affinity with that of Emmanuel Levinas, at least on some crucial issues, according to Zygmunt Bauman (1984), a philosopher within the phenomenological and postmodern tradition (Logstrup, 1997, p. xxxiii). Levinas acknowledges a fundamental metaphysical moral position to life as a face-to-face confrontation with the Other (in which I discover both my own inadequacies and my unlimited responsibility for the Other). This position reflects the infinity of mystery of the human soul. "The face of a neighbor signifies for me an exceptionable responsibility preceding every free consent, every pact, every contract" (Fink & MacIntyre, 1997).

It is suggested that what Levinas characterizes as command is close to what Logstrup speaks of as demand. According to Fink and MacIntyre's Introduction to Logstrup's *The Ethical Demand* (1997, p. xxxiv), there are at least three central features of congruence between Levinas' command and what Logstrup refers to as a demand:

❋ "My responsibility for the Other is prior to and independent of my own choices, desires and attitudes, and of my particular social relationship to the Other. It is the Other as Other, as human being . . . for whom I am responsible;

❋ This responsibility is not limited in the way in which the responsibilities . . . are presented. It is not possible to say in advance what may or may not be required of me, if I am to respond to this demand/command;

❋ This Belonging and responsibility for other is not derivable from or founded upon any universal rule or set of rights or determinate conception of the human good. For it is more fundamental in the moral life than any of these" [rules, principles].

As Fink and MacIntyre summarize, both Logstrup and Levinas are acknowledging an "experience in each of us to which we may have been blind, to which we may indeed have deliberately blinded ourselves" (Fink & MacIntyre, 1997, p. xxxiv). When one enters into a model of Caring Science, which is grounded in such fundamental realities of our life as given to us, we can no longer *turn our face away.*

In this evolving model of Caring Science, then, we dwell in this kind of holy, sacred space for our humanity, our science, our experiences, and our expressions of life and all its vicissitudes: the good, the bad, the ugly, and the holy and profane, the sovereign, the evolving consciousness toward Cosmic Love, all as sacred living entities that are given to us as learnings, lessons, teachings, beyond our control. It is through the sovereign nature of these more positive dimensions of our Belonging, Being, and Becoming that we submit to a Caring Science framework for caring-healing practices and research.

HOLDING OTHER IN OUR HANDS: LOGSTRUP'S SILENT DEMAND

Logstrup bases his ethical demand upon the fact that a characteristic of human life is a natural trust; otherwise we simply would not be able to live, and we could hardly exist if this were otherwise.

trust brings with it *laying oneself open*; with this comes
⌐selves vulnerable and brings with it self-surrender that is a
⌐c part of human life. This perspective is closely tied to caring, in
that to extend one's caring to Other is to make oneself vulnerable.
Indeed, I once heard a definition of caring as "the ability to make
oneself vulnerable. If we do not allow ourselves to be vulnerable, we are
not human. And Levinas' and Logstrup's philosophies and Caring
Science alike engage the deeply human dimensions of existence, which
seek to sustain and extend our humanity, not diminish it.

Logstrup reminds us that the basic character of trust is revealed
also in the notion of Love. This is true in Caring Science in that Caring
and Love ultimately become one. This is true in the cosmic sense due to
the fact that we are called to care, and it is through the energy of Love
that we reach out to the universe of possibilities to connect with Other,
nature, and that which is greater and more magnificent than our
isolated separate, physical-ego existence alone.

Indeed, within the context of Caring Science and this deeper
philosophical foundation, the separate ego-centered person surrenders
him/herself by going out of self, of placing something of one's own life
into the hands of the other person. This is the basis of trust, caring, and
love. These expressions are meant both metaphorically and literally. As
Logstrup put it: "we undertake an action which amounts to a delivering
of ourselves over into his hand. This self-surrender, whatever form it
may take . . . means that the self-exposure, through the trust (and
caring) . . . consists in one's having risked the chance of being rejected"
(Logstrup, 1997, p. 17). This risk-taking means that in "every human
encounter between human beings there is an unarticulated demand . . .
it always involves the risk of one person daring to lay him or herself
open to the other in the hope of a response." Logstrup indicates this fact
is the fundamental phenomenon of ethical life (p. 17). Because of this
reality, "our existence demands of us that we protect the life of the
person who has placed his or her trust in us" (p. 17). Furthermore, in
this context, trust (and caring) is revealed as "not of our own making; it
is given. Our life is so constituted that it cannot be lived except as one
person lays him or herself open to another person and puts her or
himself into that person's hands . . . " (Logstrup, 1997, p. 18).

To quote Logstrup (1997, p. 18):

> By our very attitude to one another we help to shape one
> another's world. By our attitude to the other person we help to
> determine the scope and hue of his or her world; we make it large
> or small, bright or drab, rich or dull, threatening or secure. We
> help to shape his or her world not by theories and views but by
> our very attitude toward him or her. Herein lies the unarticulated

and one might say anonymous demand that we take care of the
life which trust has placed in our hands (my italics).

Logstrup acknowledges that the ethical demand implicit in every encounter between persons is not vocal but is, and remains, silent. This demand is implied by the fact that a person "belongs to the world in which the other person has his or her life, and therefore holds something of that person's life in his or her hands" (p. 22). It is, therefore, "a demand to take care of that person's life" (p. 22).

Such a dramatic perspective has direct relevance to professions involved in caring-healing work, in that the silent demand is often the presenting "problem" in a health encounter and there is a situation for a human-to-human relationship to reveal and manifest itself most dramatically in both the Levinasian and Logstrupian sense. However, a reaching out to another in his or her vulnerability also involves making one's self vulnerable, but to do otherwise, *to turn one's face away, to not acknowledge that we are holding the life of another in our hands, can be an act of cruelty.*

It is in health care encounters that we metaphorically and otherwise hold the other person's life "in our hands," or it is "delivered over to us" (Logstrup, 1997, p. 25). However, Logstrup attempts to make clear that a person does not directly surrender his or her individuality. For example, he points out that while we are one another's world, that does not mean that we hold another person's will in our hands. "We cannot intrude upon his or her individuality and will, upon his or her personhood, in the same way that we can affect his or her emotions and in some instances even his or her destiny" (Logstrup, 1997, p. 26). Indeed, he points out this ethical demand is "a demand that we use the surrender out of which the demand has come in such a way as to free the other person from his or her confinement and to give his or her vision the widest possible horizon" (Logstrup, 1997, p. 27). Finally, he points out that responsibility for the other person in the sense that he uses it by acknowledging our inescapable dependency upon one another "never consists in our assuming the responsibility which is his or hers" (p. 28). These metaphysical moral positions from a broader and deeper philosophical context become essential when trying to explicate a Science of Caring that invites a reunion of science and metaphysics.

SUMMARY OF THE METAPHYSICAL FOUNDATION OF CARING SCIENCE AS SACRED SCIENCE

Drawing upon the wisdom and insights of the ethical and philosophical views of Levinas and Logstrup, combined with insights and discoveries among scholars in Caring theory and Unitary Sciences inquiries, we can posit the following metaphysical summary points, which seek to unite science and metaphysics. Further, these points orient Caring Science toward Sacred Science by acknowledging:

❋ The Infinity of the Human Spirit;

❋ The ancient and emerging cosmology of a unity consciousness of universal relatedness of All;

❋ The ontological ethic of *"Belong before Being"* (Levinas);

❋ The moral position of *"Facing our own and Others' Humanity"* as The Ethic for Caring, and the First Principle, for sustaining the infinity and mystery of the human condition and humanity across time (Levinas);

❋ The ethical demand that acknowledges that we *"hold another person in our hands; That there is a sovereign expression of life as given to us, before and beyond our control, with expressions of e.g. trust, love, caring, honesty, forgiveness, gratitude, and so on, beyond ego fixations and obsessive feelings that are negative expressions of life"* (Logstrup);

❋ The relationship between our consciousness, our words, and thoughts and how they positively or negatively affect our energetic-transpersonal field of Being, Becoming, and Belonging;

❋ The experienced reality that acknowledges our Caring Ethic of *Belonging and Connectedness* to the universal field of infinity, with its sovereign expression of *Love.* This ethical demand to honor the gift of life and its sovereign call to expression and engagement with other is beyond ego; it is here through engaged facing of self and other we touch and mirror the infinity of the human soul; thereby we yield to the cosmic connection between Caring/caritas and Love (Logstrup, Levinas, and Watson—see Watson Website regarding carative/caritas/love: www.uchsc.edu/nursing/caring);

❋ *Belonging and Infinite Universal-Cosmic Love* then become the First Principle and Metaphysical-Moral foundation for Caring Science. This acknowledged reality becomes the link between transpersonal energy, spirit, and the universal field of Cosmic Love that underlies the whole of life, humanity, nature, and the natural healing processes.

These dimensions are revealed as Sovereign Expressions of Life; they are given to us as gift and help to sustain humanity through our caring and healing relational processes. These views are not too unlike

Nightingale's view of natural healing process and draw upon the spiritual dimensions that are the greatest source of healing. In acknowledging and honoring our relationship with this greater than our control process for caring and healing and our science for these phenomena, we as health professionals become part of the mystery of the great circle of living and dying; we participate, co-participate with this evolving pattern that is greater than ourselves and our control, across time, space, and physicality.

> We did not create it, something is given prior to and as a precondition of all that we may think and do; a recognition that this experience and reality to which we may have been blind, to which we may indeed have deliberately blinded ourselves (Logstrup, 1997, p. xxxv).

Conceptual Commonalities of Transpersonal Caring (TC)–Unitary Science (US) and Metaphysical Foundation of Levinas' and Logstrup's Philosophy

❊ Both TC and US reside within a unitary-transformative framework, honoring the universal oneness and connectedness of all. This integration is consistent with Levinas' notion of Infinity and Logstrup's view that our life is not of our own making. We did not create it . . . "My life has taken me over before I have taken my life over."

❊ Both TC and US integrate principles of energy and resonancy with caring consciousness. Integrating principles of resonancy into caring consciousness and caring field is congruent with Levinas' notion of relationship and sustaining humanity at the individual and collective level; it is consistent with Logstrup's notion that we hold another person's life in our hands, and this primordial fact manifests in a caring moment, any and all presenting human-to-human encounter; we make a difference with our sovereign expressions and attitudes of life that are beyond ego and self-cause;

❊ Both TC and US make explicit a relational ontology; thus caring, as relational, is acknowledged as an ethical-moral foundation for science. Having caring as moral foundation is congruent with Levinas' notion of Ethics as first philosophy and introduces metaphysics into science; the relational aspect in Logstrup's work is evident in his ethical demand as acknowledging the fact that we cannot help being dependent upon each other as a basic condition for human existence;

❈ Both TC and US make explicit an expanded view of what it means to be human and to sustain humanity—acknowledging the unitary, transpersonal, evolving nature of humankind, both immanent and transcendent. This view is consistent with Levinas' notion of Belonging before Being as part of humanity and its existence and relates to Logstrup's ethical demand of "inescapably up to me what I do with those parts of the other person's lives that are in my power. I can take care of and help the other to the best of my ability or else ignore or even destroy what has been delivered into my hands (Logstrup, 1997, p. xxix);

❈ Both TC and US make connections between energy field and its continuous, infinite notion, connecting with the mystery, the infinity, the universal field. This makes explicit connection of congruence with Levinas' view of "Ethics of Face" in that we are connected with mystery of infinity of the soul when facing another; this notion relates to Logstrup's notion that our life is not of our own making—something is given prior to and as a precondition of all;

❈ This emerging cosmology for Caring Science is considered a primordial precondition of life and Caring; that is, the evolving notion of Cosmic Love as the highest level of Caring Consciousness communicates and connects with a deep, abiding spirit-filled energy that permeates, enfolds, and envelops all of life as the universal energy, which sustains humanity and nature across all time.

❈ Different Health Disciplines, e.g., Nursing, Medicine, Biomedical science explorations, Mind-Body medicine, Healing professions in general, (consciously and unconsciously) can and are moving toward this cosmology as part of their evolution and transcendence of conventional, separate, medicalized views of science and caring-healing practices; what is emerging is a framework of expanding consciousness consistent with Caring Science.

By integrating evolving consciousness with Caring and Love along with transpersonal and unitary views expanded by Levinas and Logstrup, we can affirm a deep ethical-ontology of relation and spirit that transcends duality; thus, we uncover the moral-metaphysical foundation for Caring Science. This integration of infinity, evolving consciousness with Love and spirit, invites the sacred (holy) and mystery of life to return to our profession and our healing practices.

9

Caring and Science

A Contemporary
Orientation

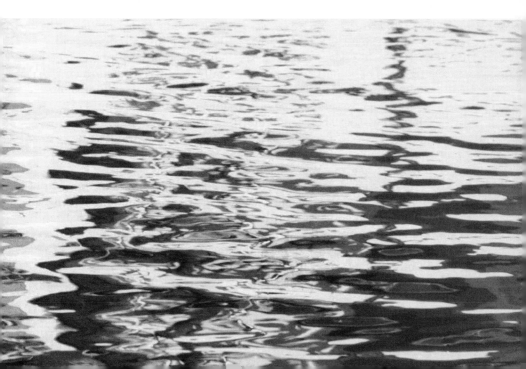

There is growing awareness that as clinical care issues accelerate, issues about facing and sustaining our humanity, and the human-to-human connections and relationships, become moral acts. They precede clinical knowledge. Simultaneously there is the demand for knowledge and practices that attend to these moral and metaphysical realities of non-physical, non-local, energetic fields, and relational infinite phenomena in healing and treatment outcomes. This momentum is beginning to dominate some of the scientific developments and discourse of this day. One of the dominant debates is related to whether a discipline (that is the knowledge boundaries, the underlying philosophies, values, ethic, research patterns and traditions) should inform a profession (the practices and use of the disciplinary knowledge in the field) or whether professional issues guide the direction of a discipline.

In this instance, consider Caring as an underlying disciplinary philosophical, theoretical base encompassing value, ethic, and growing empirical knowledge that can and must be included into our professional practices. A Caring Science orientation comes into play as necessary for survival of health professionals, to sustain the humanity of the practitioners, as well as to cultivate and create new scientific and humane systems for healing. Caring Science can serve as a guide for not only nursing but also all health professions into a common disciplinary matrix for entering into this new unknown scientific territory.

Knowledge is not diminished in this model, it is initiated; it enters into new territory informed by the values of being human, which actually comes before knowledge; indeed Caring Science, which embraces *The Ethics of Face and acknowledgement "We hold Other in our hands,"* is a moral act and shapes and informs the knowledge we use. Thus, a Caring Science framework helps us both morally and metaphysically, both personally and professionally, to address the growing old/new phenomena related to healing while not ignoring mainstream scientific-technological developments and needs.

In nursing, there has been ambiguity about which informed the other: that is, does the discipline inform the profession? Or does the profession, with all its immediacy of practice demands of doing, inform the nature of its science? Whereas historically the practice, politics, controls, and system demands dictated the educational and research traditions for early nursing science, what remains is an ambiguity with respect to what and which informs which, and why one or the other direction may be the desired starting point to offer mature disciplinary status and balance (in actuality, they inform or should inform each other).

Simultaneously and paradoxically, as part of its maturity and coming of age as a discipline, nursing (or at least a subset of the nursing discipline) has been silently behind the scenes of mainstream science, clarifying and questioning its disciplinary values, goals, philosophies, theories, and ethics, along with the underlying knowledge base that guides professional practice. This questioning has led more and more to a hopeful paradigm for science and practice, which more closely mirrors the human relational phenomena of caring and healing and the new foci and expanded views of what counts as knowledge, both physical-material as well as well as non-physical. The paradigm that is emergent in this work on Caring Science serves as a moral, metaphysical, and scientific foundation for nursing and all health sciences.

PROFESSIONAL REMEMBERING

It seems that somewhere along the way we have forgotten that one of the greatest honors and privileges one can have is to be able to care for another person. Such personal, intimate connections and relations touch on the Holy, as well as the horrific at times. Caring is such a vulnerable place; first, because we come face to face with our own humanity and ourselves. In this place, we realize that one person's level of humanity reflects back on the other. The other reason this place of caring and healing transcends traditional medical thinking and science is because, when we locate ourselves in this new space, we are *remembering* our own and others' humanity and our shared belonging to the infinity of universal field of love that embraces spirit. We are *remembering* we are touching the life force, the very soul of another person, hence ourselves.

Logstrup (1997) in his use of the Hand metaphor *reminded* us that morally and metaphysically, if not scientifically, in this field of caring-healing work, we literally and metaphorically *hold another person in our hands*. Whereas Levinas helps us *remember* to Face our humanity by honoring our Belonging to Infinity and mystery of whole, Logstrup helps us *remember* that we hold another's life in our hands and our life is given to us as a gift with its sovereign expressions of trust, love, and deeper emotions beyond our control.

Logstrup's moral, and perhaps sacred, reminder is that "Life has been given to us. We have not ourselves created it" (Logstrup, 1997, p. 19). And within this framework, we realize that "either we take care of the other person's life or we ruin it" (Logstrup, 1997, p. 18). He explores this deeply profound meaning for life by his statement, " the demand is implied by the very fact that a person belongs to the world in which the other person has his or her life, and therefore holds something of that person's life in his or her hands, it is therefore a demand to take care of that person's life" (Logstrup, 1997, p. 22).

Logstrup points out that to "have something in one's hand" is a metaphor (p. 28). This endows the metaphor with a certain emotional power. "The emotional significance of the metaphor grows out of the contrast in the relationship to which it refers, namely, that we have the power to determine the direction of something in another person's life . . . or his or her entire destiny" (p. 28). This kind of thinking parallels the concept of a caring moment (Watson, 1988, 1999a,b) whereby a caring moment as a transpersonal event has been defined as:

❋ *"A transpersonal caring relationship connotes a spirit to spirit unitary connection within a caring moment, honoring the embodied spirit of both* (Watson, 2002, p. 458);

❋ *A transpersonal caring moment transcends the ego level of both . . . creating a caring field with new possibilities of how to be in the moment* (Watson, 2002, p. 458);

❋ *'. . . the process goes beyond itself, and becomes part of the life history of each person, as well as part of the larger, deeper complex pattern of life'"* (Watson, 1988, p. 59).

There is an intersection between and among the caring moment, transpersonal caring theory, and relationships with both Levinas' and Logstrup's philosophical-moral-metaphysical positions. The notions of "making a difference," in a moment, for better or for worse in another's life, is integral to the Caring theory framework as well as Levinas' Ethic of Face and Logstrup's notion of Holding another's life in one's hands in the moment of encounter. Further congruence is found between the notion of connecting with Infinity, the soul, and mystery of life and human-universe oneness of Belonging before individual Being. New connections become more explicit between Caring and Love as part of the infinity of Universal life force-energy of the universe.

Levinas' (1969) philosophy of Totality and Infinity captures this deeply and poignantly for science and philosophy and offers us an ethic of relating with the infinity and mystery of the human soul, placing our humanity within the larger universe. Likewise, Logstrup's (1997) work adds additional philosophical-ethical confirmation for this foundational moral-metaphysical perspective for Caring Science.

However, the gap in nursing science, which lingers into this new millennium, in spite of amazing progress, is the fact that nursing science is still largely modeled from a non-human science model for its disciplinary foundation for professional practice, thus separating the practitioner's world from the world of science. Thus, all health professions at this time are largely still forced to succumb to either a professional world orientation, without a disciplinary meta-narrative to guide them, or to a detached scientific orientation. However, a Caring Science disciplinary matrix can inform our scientific phenomena and practice demands alike. Once Caring is placed within a discipline's frame of reference for its science, it automatically helps to solve some of the lingering ethical, philosophical, and humane issues for caring-healing science and practices that touch the human mind, heart, and soul of humanity itself.

In this process of redefining science to embrace the infinity of humanity itself, we realize that our jobs and our science have been too small and limited with respect to honoring the deeply human nature of caring-healing practices. For Nightingale, nursing involved a sense of presence higher than the human, "a divine intelligence that creates, sustains, and organizes the universe—and our awareness of an inner connection with this higher reality" (Macrae, 1995, 2001). She pointed out that the care of the soul could never be separated from that of the body. She was very clear that nursing, and we might now say all healing practice, is a spiritual practice and a human service connecting us with something greater than ourselves. Perhaps now the infinity of the human soul, as put forth by Levinas, forces us to "face our humanity," which is beyond the physical face alone, a moral invitation responsibility to engage and respond to the infinite that we are all apart of.

WORKING DEFINITION OF CARING SCIENCE

Caring Science has been described as "an evolving philosophical-ethical-epistemic field of study that is grounded in the discipline of nursing and informed by related fields" (Watson & Smith, 2002, p. 456). While many nursing scholars consider Caring as one central feature within the meta-paradigm of nursing knowledge and practices (Watson & Smith, 2002), it is now posited as a foundational disciplinary framework for all caring-healing professions, moving beyond nursing.

What is unique about Caring Science is in making it explicit, that as soon as one places Caring within its science model, or as soon as one locates the Science model within the context of Caring Ontology (which is relational), science automatically grounds itself in, and has responsibility to, attend to an ethical-moral-metaphysical stance. Caring forces us as individuals and professions to *Face our relation* of infinite responsibility of *Belonging* to other human beings as well as to a unitary field of all-our-relations. Such an orientation becomes non-dualistic, relational, and unified, wherein there is connectedness of all. Newman, Sime, and Corcoran-Perry (1991) refers to this as a unitary transformative paradigm; it has also been referred to as non-local consciousness and Era III thinking (Dossey, 1991, 1993; Watson, 1999b). Caring Science intersects with arts and humanities and related fields of study and practices, including, for example, eco-caring, peace studies, philosophy-ethics, women/feminist studies, theology, education, and mind-body-spirit medicine/nursing and the growing field of complementary medicine, health, and healing (Watson & Smith, 2002).

In some instances in the nursing literature, caring has been specifically tied to healing and part of the paradigmatic foundation for the discipline of nursing. Even more foundational, caring has been described as a sacred art, which calls this work into a deeper life, a communion with the other, moving us forward, whereby we honor the fundamental sacredness and unity of all of life (Watson, 1995, p. 67). Indeed, some caring scholars have posited that Caring is sometimes, if not always, an act of Love (Reason, 1993; Swanson, 1990; Watson, 1988, 1999, 2003).

10

Caring Science as Disciplinary Foundation for Health Sciences

What about a science model that inspires, captures, embraces and contains the heart and hands as well as the mind? A model that faces the infinity of the human spirit, the over-soul of life, as the cosmic union that connects rather than separates us? A model that honors the awe, wonder, beauty, mystery, miracles of humankind and all living-non-living existence. Can we envision a science model that unites us to this great unknown that holds us in its hand, when we do not know the way, and are called to surrender to the sovereign expressions of life that emanate from the gift of life itself, and draw us to them? Not only during turmoil, sickness, despair, suffering and angst, but also during joy, bliss, quiet, peace . . . reminding us that these are all given to us as possibilities, as openings to the transcendence of deep Love/Caritas, the cosmic energy of the universe which radiates with and from our open heart, releasing vibratory Love energy into the universe and all our relations!.

JW Bahia, Sea of Cortez, México, February, 2003

In embarking upon a model of Caring Science, we create new open space to allow such phenomena of heart, hands, and the Infinity of the human soul and Cosmic Love as the highest level of consciousness to be acknowledged, as part of our evolving humanity; as part of an evolving human science that opens the door to metaphysics of Caring/ *Caritas* as a supreme life force, our foundation of grace, mercy, and blessings in our Belonging-Being-Knowing-Doing that is the deep source of all true knowing, living, being, and healing.

In Caring Science, we allow for the inner and infinite nature of our reality of Belonging and Being. We are not restricted to the outer, physical world alone, which is the science model of a past era, which cuts our humanity off from its life source—the human spirit and our Originary primordial Love; the Love that Levinas (1969) discussed as an "Ethic as First Principle," which comes before ontology. As Levinas put it: "this is not meant to be anti-intellectual; rather . . . . In distinguishing between the objectifying act and the metaphysical we are on our way not to the denunciation of intellectualism but to its very . . . development" (Levinas, 1969, p. 109). So, perhaps the rhetorical question for our evolving science is: can it contain an underlying metaphysical-philosophical-ethical foundation for its essence and its existence . . . for its *das Sein?* * Or must we revert to and continue to succumb to classic assumptions of science for our human phenomena, which objectifies humans and keeps our knowledge limited in time and space and

das Sein, the German term used by Heidegger, denoting and further explicating the concept of Being as existence, or Being for itself alone (Heidegger, 1959, p. 54).

physicality? The purpose here is to consciously evolve, recognizing and acknowledging that information is not necessarily knowledge; knowledge is not understanding; understanding is not wisdom. It is an evolutionary process of awakening to the differences, seeking movement toward wisdom and integration of whole.

As we examine our truth of Belonging—Being, Knowing, and Doing our caring-healing work in the world—how can we any longer bear to sustain and perpetuate an empty, hollow model, especially once we honor and acknowledge our participation with the infinity and mystery of healing and life itself? This evolving model of Caring Science opens science and our knowing to its Source—not its separation—from the knowable and the unknowable and to a wisdom that knows/honors/surrenders to the differences.

Some assumptions between Caring and Love are already noted in the Caring literature. For example (Adapted from Watson, 1988, 1999, p. 32):

✼ Caring and love are the most universal, the most tremendous, and the most mysterious of cosmic forces: they comprise the primal and universal psychic energy;

✼ Often these needs and realities are overlooked; or we know people need each other in loving and caring ways, but often we do not behave well toward each other. If our humanness is to survive, however, we need to become more caring and loving to nourish our humanity and evolve as a civilization and live together;

✼ As a beginning we have to impose our own will to care and love upon our own behavior and not on others. We have to treat our self with love, gentleness, and dignity before we can respect and care for others with love, gentleness, and dignity;

✼ Human caring can be effectively demonstrated and practiced only interpersonally. The intersubjective human process keeps alive a common sense of humanity; it teaches us how to be more human by identifying ourselves with others, whereby the humanity of one is reflected in the other. (This perspective does not preclude non-physical caring connections emerging through authentic virtual caring connections, which remain as interpersonal, for example: "higher frequency thoughts such as love and caring, even communicated from a distance, carry higher frequency energy into space; the other has energetic access to the experience that has been communicated to them, even virtually." [See Watson, 2002, *IJHC,* for more on this point]);

❋ Health professionals' social, moral, and scientific contributions to humankind and civilization lie in their commitment to sustain human caring ideals in theory, practice, research, and education.

These assumptions put forth in 1985 (Watson, 1985, reprinted, 1988, 1999) have a striking resemblance to the philosophies and metaphysics of both Levinas and Logstrup; for example, with respect to the:

❋ Notions of primordial Love as originary and infinite;

❋ The necessity of honoring our connections and with Others to sustain our own and others' humanity;

❋ And the role of caring and Love as critical to our evolving humanity and survival as a human civilization;

❋ Honoring the reality that a human-to-human encounter, one with another, whereby we *face our shared humanity,* is an ethical event we cannot turn our face away from;

❋ Acknowledgement of moral-metaphysical foundation for our work in the world of science and practice alike.

Caring Science, then, helps to frame and claim our Values and deep longings that call each of us to remember why we are here and why we came to do this work at this time in the world. We pause here to ponder the lyrics of John Astin (1991).

Why have you come to earth?
Do you remember . . . ?
Why have you taken birth?
Why have you come?
To love, serve, and remember.

11

Professional/ Personal Remembering

Perhaps I am here to *remember,* remind myself and others that it is our humanity that both wounds us and heals us and those whom we serve; and as W.H. Auden helps us remember: *in the end, it is only Love that truly matters* for this deeply human and humane work, which cries out for a new model of science. It is in entering into and participating with the great mysteries of the sacred circle of life and death and our surrender to why we came here that we engage in true healing. It is in attending to, honoring, entering into, connecting with our deep humanity, we find the ethic and artistry of Belonging, Being, Loving, and Caring that sustains and transcends simultaneously. We are not machines, as we have been conditioned, but spirit made whole.

PERSONAL REMEMBERING

In 1997, I was faced with a life-changing event in which I experienced Cosmic love, and I cannot turn back. It occurred when I had to lie still 24 hours a day, on a massage table, with my head in the cradle; I had a 15-minute break each hour; otherwise I had to keep my head down, for almost 3 months. Even when I was able to have more time "up," I still had to keep my head down. All of this was required because of a traumatic eye injury, an uncanny accident in which I was hit by a golf club, accidentally getting into the line of fire of my little 9-year-old grandson at the time.

During this time, I also had to have silence and inner quiet, so as not to disturb my eye and its sacred healing process. My husband and I, along with my family and close friends, created sacred space for my needs; we ritualized all of my experience by not allowing negative energy into my room; through practice of meditation; through ritual of removing shoes; through rituals of listening to healing music and sounds; through my husband reading me literature, love stories, and reciting poetry—I particularly remember W.H. Auden's lines from *As I Walked Out One Evening;* he read again and again to me, and I tried to memorize parts of it that were so beautiful, loving, and touching, such as the following lines:

" . . . Love has no ending.
I'll love you dear, I'll love you
Till China and Africa meet,
And the river jumps over the mountain
And the salmon sing in the street.
I'll love you till the ocean
Is folded and hung up to dry,
And the seven stars go squawking
Like geese about the sky . . .

O look, look in the mirror?
O look in your distress:
Life remains a blessing . . . .
(W.H. Auden, As I Walked Out One Evening).

During this time, we expressed our deep, deep love and devotion for each other and our awe at being together with such love, appreciating each other and life, more than ever. We ritualized my healing through his giving me massages (in spite of being an attorney, he also was very avant-garde: he learned massage at Esalen, was a practitioner of Vipassana meditation, wrote poetry; knew music, literature, and art and used it throughout this time). We ritualized my healing through having special time with my grandson who read to me and with whom we created sacred rituals for both of our shared healing, by drawing mandalas, by reading Annie Dillard, revealing the sacredness and beauty of nature, which was of great interest to him at the time; through my quiet practice of paying attention to simple things: the way the light came into my room; the color, fragrance, and texture of the roses; outside nature and the subtle changes of season outside my treetop window from my second-story bedroom window. I quietly watched the changing birdlife and aspen leaves changing from spring, summer, into autumn—seeing with wonder, upside down, as it were, as if I had never seen before, so grateful for the gift of sight and quiet, suspended in a bubble of total love.

Then, there were my special friends and colleagues doing loving therapeutic touch on a regular basis. (My gratitude continues for Dr. Janet Quinn, my primary loving Therapeutic Touch [TT] practitioner; Marilyn Fogerty for her rainbow drop massages, foot massages; and Beverly Lyne for her intermittent TT sessions and other gifts of love and comfort when needed; the frequent loving, concerned calls from Meditation master teacher, Shinzen Young, who telephoned my husband and me and did meditations for us on our speaker phone, since I could neither stand nor sit up. Of course, my abiding gratitude to all my friends and colleagues who prayed for me, who sent meals, lattes, flowers, cards, gifts, and healing objects to sustain me, and whom I could not reciprocate even through writing; I had to learn to accept unconditional giving of love, without expectation of having it returned by me in some physical manifestation, violating customary norms, (which was a lesson in itself.).

During this entire experience, every day, my husband and I would ritualize and honor the love we were receiving by setting aside a special private, intimate time: This consisted of my husband opening each card, one by one, reading the message and crying from the sweet experience of receiving love and healing thoughts from others. He would then pass the card to me for me to try to see, even though lying on my stomach. This was a very healing act and with each card I realized how much love I/we were receiving; I felt a deep abiding love that held me/us in grace and mercy, even in the midst of deep angst around saving or losing my eye, my sight, and my way of being to date. In spite of or because of it all, I felt a deep peace, Love, and trust in the midst of despair. I surrendered to what was whole and holy for me/us.

Through all of these experiences and more, I was becoming more contemplative, accepting, allowing an inner stillness to emerge. I was allowing myself to feel a gentleness and deep kindness toward myself in order to honor the sacredness of my eye's healing; I honored the injury and the whole experience as a lesson for stopping long enough to allow my soul and deep self to catch up with me, after busy, active, non-stop, intense work life and travel.

As a result of this tragic-trauma-blessing-gift (depending upon how one perceives), I learned to be still; I learned to receive; I learned to surrender; I learned to feel love both inside and out; I learned to accept and see/feel all the beauty, simplicity, wonders, depth of life around me, even the grain in the wood of the hardwood floors in my bedroom; I experienced this even in the midst of despair and acute, indescribable pain; I became contemplative to the extent that I had mystical experiences, heard voices, and had deep Biblical dreams, about approaching the holy, of life and love being opened unto me. Tolle has noted that in such an experience when the mind is still and needs to be still, there is much more to see, hear that often "cannot be named, something ineffable, some deep, inner holy essence" (Tolle, 1999, p. 80). That helps to describe my experience, beyond words, but profound sense of being present in the now, waiting, still but alert, open, expressing a state of consciousness described by mystics.

In other words, at another level, I had the gift of being the recipient of my own theory, of experiencing a Caring Science in practice. This was epitomized through my husband's taking care of me as a spiritual practice, with a loving devotion—one of the greatest gifts of my life (yet one of the greatest pains and mysteries of life, which will be explained later). Indeed, at one point when he was giving me a massage, he exclaimed seemingly "out of the blue": *"I feel like I have been preparing all my life, just for this, to be here and take care of you now."* I shall never forget those words, as they resonate later in my experience for deeper meanings. Those who already know, and have read about my story, are already tuned into the belated significance and powerful meaning of his words, which I will explain later.

But for now, I want to explain that all of this experience and time out/in resulted in one epiphany of a moment, when I had this powerful cosmic moment when I felt that I had *Become Love!* It was not a feeling of *being* loved, or being *in* love, I felt *I WAS LOVE,* and it was as if I realized that was what I had come here to remember. I felt an *AT-ONE-MENT* with all. I experienced what Whitehead called *"the eternal now,"* a full presence that transcended any sense of ordinary time; was timeless and eternal in the moment. I now believe my experience of *Becoming Love* is our true state of Belonging-Being-Becoming that we are all seeking to remember in our own way. I felt I had received a holy gift, which I cannot forget.

Although I could not stay there, have not been able to stay there in that Cosmic space and place, I long to return to it; and I could not/cannot forget that I experienced it. Indeed, I am now more attuned to when I am not in right relation with this new center of inner quiet. Once experienced, it is a gift beyond gifts and one that now guides my life and my *remembering.*

Now that I have once experienced and am *remembering* such a profound and prophetic gift, it is known as a truth that cannot be denied; however, now my lesson/learning/human task is to more fully and constantly cultivate this reality as a living process for my Belonging-Being-Becoming more and more human and humane by feeling more and more Caring and Loving flowing through me, not from me. I now feel this pull, both personally and professionally, and yes, even scientifically, to integrate this *remembering, this new reality,* we most often are not awakened to. Both Logstrup and Levinas also are trying to help us see that there is an experience in each of us to which we may have been blind, to which we may indeed have deliberately blinded ourselves (Fink & MacIntyre, 1997, p. xxxv). It is as if through my accident, which blinded me in one eye, I am learning to see that which is a deeper level of seeing. So I continue to teach, to write about, to try to live that which I now *see* and yet still need to learn the most about—as perhaps which remains true for all of us on this path and earth-plane's journey.

It is through us *facing ourselves,* and the depths of the dark and light sides of our souls in such circumstances, that we likewise touch the depths of each other in our shared humanity, that perhaps then and only then do we learn to *see again!* We discover the pain and joy side by side, and we can hold them both simultaneously for we hold a new vision of self, other, and life itself.

I was alone in my journey toward healing, but I was never alone. The love and caring and the human presence of those who surrounded and protected me, both near and afar, sustained me. It was the human-to-human event, even though I could not hold my head up, that I still experienced the mystery and wonder of *soul-to-soul* connections through our *facing* and deepening our humanity in this particular situation and life circumstance. I also realized that others were vicariously responding with me in my experience, and in giving out love and prayers and caring-healing thoughts to me, they were also filling themselves up with love and healing, because of the mutuality of our human connection.

FACING OUR HUMANITY

To return to Levinas' notion of facing our humanity, we find that one person's story may be any of our stories as we face ourself; thus "one face" mirrors the oneness of human experience. This view intersects with and is revealed through ancient poetic words of Rumi.

In Rumi's *The Glance,* the experience when eyes meet becomes a reminder of how we mirror the human soul, through the eyes, the look, and the glance. In Rumi's words:

> I see my beauty in you. I become a mirror that cannot close its eyes to your longing . . . . These thousands of worlds that arise from nowhere, how does your face contain them? . . . Out of eternity (infinity) I turn my face to you and into eternity.
>
> Rumi, 2001b, p. 12

According to Levinas, in the encounter with other, with the face, we have the primary event of being. "Meaning is the Face of the other, and all recourse to words takes place already within the primordial face-to-face language" (Levinas, 1969, p. 206). More specifically, Levinas' notion of Ethics of Face, "In openness to the human Face, the human being, being addressed by its vulnerability, by its 'nudity', a moral responsibility sets the scene. The ethical event of encountering the other, breaks with ontology and being for itself alone" (Levinas, 1969, p. 200).

It can be put this way: "A look, a glance, a gaze, a touch, a voice, which invites and welcomes. A Face which connects with the infinity of humanity itself, rather than a turning away, is beyond clinical" (Nortvedt, 2000, p. 6); it is entering into humanity itself and the infinity of the universe; it touches cosmic Love. The artistic sensitivity to being human, in *facing* our own and another's humanity in reaching out to Other, is a healing act itself. It takes place in any caring moment where there is an authentic human-to-human encounter, engagement, spirit-to-spirit, soul-to-soul...face-to-face (Watson, 1999b). This thesis grounds the ethics, the artistry, and science of being human; such a view sets the scene for moral responsibility for our science. Caring Science acknowledges and opens to these primordial face-to-face realities of Belonging and Being in relation with life and the infinity of the universe.

Such a basic foundation for caring and healing awakens human values, human compassion, caring and humane responses that allow us to face our own and another's humanity. This view of science is in no way antithetical to knowledge. Rather, the moral, metaphysical, and artistic view of life precedes knowledge in the sense of being prior to it and welcoming it. In Levinas' view, the encounter with the Other is the signification; the Other is an event of particularity, his or her hurt, vulnerability, pain, grief, suffering, and so on; elicits a human-to-human universal response that links back to the infinite. Such a view of knowledge of Caring and Face as proposed here becomes what Nortvedt calls the *"Primordial core"* of clinical knowledge and care practices.

Caring Science within this contemporary philosophical-ethical framework allows us to birth a new era as science "enters yet another phase of its journey" (Swimme, 1996, p. x); no longer simply a materialistic study of reality, but allowing for exploration of the evolving human and our unity with the universe—a scientific cosmology that restores wholeness; a science that opens, not closes, the great sacred circle of birth-life-death-rebirth. Caring science as explored here offers a moral, sacred foundation to health, healing knowledge, and practices within the human-universe relations we share.

12

Evolving Consciousness

Caring and Cosmic Love as a Universal Field

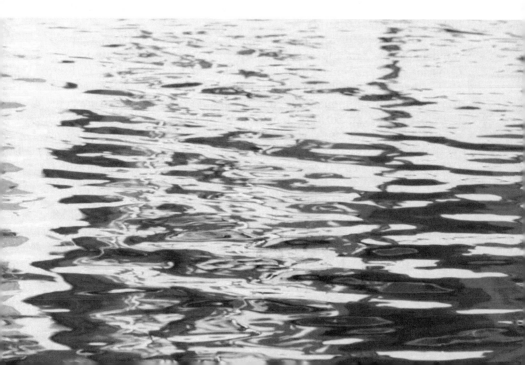

The circuit of love then becomes complete as the soul of love returns to the Source of Love. Love pours into love, races into love, expands into love and finds only love. Human love then realizes that it has always belonged completely to Divine Love.

Lex Hixon (In Vaughn, 1995, p. 105)

Love is the medicine that accelerates the process of healing. There is no other medicine but unconditional love.

Don Miguel Ruiz. 1999, p. 170

. . . Tired and in pain I searched the world for help until I found in love the cure for my pain.

Rumi, 2001a, p. 148.

Love's path is outside of all religious sects.

Rumi, 2001a, p. 46.

Within this emerging Caring Science framework, which transcends conventional health science models, I have acknowledged both philosophical and theoretical connections between Evolving Consciousness, Universal Field of Infinity of Caring, and Love. These connections have been explored and acknowledged from prominent nursing literature on Caring, as well as the philosophies, ethics, and metaphysics of Levinas and Logstrup, which remind us of our infinity of Belonging, before our individual existence; the sovereign nature of expressions of love as a gift of life, which we did not create nor control, in which we hold another in our hands.

I now turn toward a more explicit exploration of Love, as ineffable as that is, but approached as the highest level of (Caring) Consciousness, as Spirit-filled Energy, as The Universal Energy Field that surrounds all of life: a resource we draw upon as the Source. Aside from the Bible, religious texts, poetry, art, and sages across time, one of the most renowned authors to acknowledge Love in this deeper cosmic as well as scientific sense was Teilhard de Chardin (1959). He reminded us that we are accustomed to consider only the sentimental face of love, the joys and miseries it causes us (at the ego-physical level). But he too took an evolutionary, dynamic perspective to help us understand Love in a different higher/deeper sense.

He viewed Love in its fuller evolutionary sense, as well as biological reality, as the "affinity of being with being" (or we might think here of *Belonging with Infinity* in Levinas' sense). In this sense, love is not peculiar to human; it is a general property of all of life. It is that energy–force field of infinity that is the internal propensity to unite, the *within of thing* (Chardin, 1959, p. 264). He makes the case that we should assume the presence of Love in everything that is. In this "confluent ascent of consciousness" (p. 264), the fragments of the world seek each other so that the world may come to being; this is the universal gravity of bodies, which moves nature (p. 265). He viewed this notion of Love as Cosmic Energy "at the fount," a *within* of things, which goes down into the internal zone of spiritual attractions.

In Chardin's words (1959, p. 265): "Love in all its subtleties is nothing more, and nothing less, than the more or less direct trace marked on the heart of the element by the psychical convergence of the universe upon itself. This, if I am not mistaken is the ray of light which will help us to see more clearly around us."

He goes on to say that "Love alone is capable of uniting living beings in such a way as to complete and fulfill them, for it alone takes them and joins them by what is deepest in themselves" (Chardin, 1959, p. 265). With his point of view, "we may well need to imagine our power of loving developing (evolving) until it embraces the total of men (sic) and of the earth" (p. 266). This view is consistent with the evolving consciousness and connections between Love, Caring, and even Peace, whereby we may be evolving toward a moral community in which we discover and act upon the unitary perspective of our world and universe. Within this point of view, Chardin said that the universe is a collector and conservator, not of mechanical energy, as we supposed, but of persons. This perspective is not too unlike Whitehead's in that Whitehead referred to the collective past and the eternal now converging in the present when two persons come together; here we have soul-to-soul connections within a caring-healing framework that unites love, caring consciousness, and energy within a given field of union that transcends time, space, and physicality (Chardin, 1959, pp. 272–273; Watson, 1988, 1999).

In this framework of evolving consciousness, with Love being the highest level of consciousness, Chardin posits a cosmic involution, whereby our consciousness becomes co-extensive with the universe and therefore exists as a converging and evolving universe toward unification by the communicating action of Love (Chardin, 1959, p. 310).

From another perspective, Barbara Brennan and her work on energy and light bring a contemporary view on Love (1993, p. 317). On a spiritual level, we know and are told, by sages and contemporaries across time, that our choices each moment are love and fear. We know this consciously or unconsciously; it is the choice between being undefended or defended, of being connected, or separate and disconnected. The choice for Love is to let our core essence shine forth. Barbara Brennan suggests that if we can not make the choice for love in the moment, then the next choice for love is to accept our human condition as it is and work through another life lesson to gain more self-aware-ness (1993, p. 317). Part of our difficulty is that part of the human condition is such that we are unable to always choose to express our core essence; we do not know how to do so, and we are all on a learning path toward it. We have not yet learned about Cosmic, eternal Love. From Brennan's perspective, the journey toward Love is allowing our inner light to emerge from the source of our existence, our conscious-ness, our divinity.

DIVINE LOVE

To attain a sense and experience of divine love we have to give time and energy to this part of our daily lives. As Brennan indicates, it may mean meditation; it may mean regular silent sunrise walks on the beach or mountains. It may be going regularly to a religious service, poetry readings, symphony, listening to inspiration music, etc. (Brennan, 1993, p. 273). This experience is associated directly with our own self-healing efforts that transcend one's usual ego-personality driven reality, lifting us to a higher/deeper spiritual plane and exis-tence. These moments are filled with peace, beauty, and a sense of serenity, awe, and gratitude and love. As these experiences become a regular part of one's life that are cultivated and practiced on a daily basis we begin to recognize Love, both personal as well as divine/eternal/cosmic, which is holding us, surrounding us—as the deep source of life within and without. Ultimately this desire for eternal love seeks a connection with God and a desire for spiritual communion, moving beyond the ego-physical-material–centered existence.

This seeking serves as a deep inner longing, leading us toward and perhaps through our life's path at some level, journeying to fulfill our purpose for being here; helping us to *remember* who we are and why we came. This experience could be considered an inner healing moment for us. At that moment and during this time, we may consider our self whole, holy, at peace, or *At Onement*. We are in *right-relation with our self and our world;* honoring this spirit-filled relationship and deeper inner need and longing to connect with this eternal/cosmic/divine Love.

Within a framework of Caring Science, we are *reminded* once again that compassionate human service and authentic Caring are ulti-mately motivated by Love, both human and Cosmic. By attending to, honoring, entering into, connecting with our deep humanity, we find the foundation of Loving and Caring. We find the ancient truths of our work. We share the wisdom of mystics-poets-philosophers who capture the Infinity and mystery of the human soul, mirrored through the *Ethics of Face*. The fact remains that we *hold another's life in our hands.*

How can we dare to be so bold to bring Caring and Love and Infinity of Universal Energy and soul into our lives and work and world again? Because without returning to this ancient place of cosmic power, energy, beauty, and hope, we are inclined toward what Levinas referred to as a *totalizing of self and other*; that is, a congealing of our humanity, separating us from any connection with spirit, with infinity, with the Great Divine—with no hope for caring, healing, and wholeness. A totalizing occurs when there is no relational engagement, no soul connection: thus, no cosmic human field to engage and sustain our shared humanity. This totalizing of self and other, this turning away from the mystery of our shared humanity and Divine connection, can be an act of cruelty to self and others; an inhumane act toward human civilization itself, perpetuating more inhumane acts, violence, and destruction of human spirit and love in our work and world.

So rather than asking *how can we dare to bring Love and Caring together into our lives and work and our science? We can ask: How can we bear not to?*

In this view of ethics and metaphysics and metaphors of *Love, Face, and Hands,* which converge within a Caring Science context, Love becomes Originary; Primordial. Love watches over the other demands, such as justice (Nortvedt, 2001). The subject as Other is an incomprehensible, infinite Otherness. The human face is not a concept; the human heart is not a concept, it is not a figure whose message can be captured by conventional knowledge from the head. It is the Other, the face, the heart-felt call in its exposedness, its nudity, as an opening toward the infinite, the infinity of Cosmic Love that reminds us that we belong together in this life as given to us, which is beyond our control, making one responsible for the Other. It is in the Other that we see ourselves and the infinity and mystery of our own soul, reflected back to us through Other.

Within this metaphysics and science model, we begin to *remember* that we dwell in *Originary Love, Cosmic and Divine.* Such a perspective comes before and informs our clinical judgments in caring—healing, treating, curing, and so on, and in turn can serve as an ontological, epistemological, and methodological foundation for clinical care (Nortvedt, 2001).

This ethic, moral foundation, and metaphysics of Love and Caring become manifestations of both Levinas' and Logstrup's first principles, first philosophy, and underlying ethic for facing and sustaining not only humanity but also foundation for the fact that we are holding others in our hands. This awareness informs our health and healing disciplines and professions for a new science. This first principle reminds us of the sacred world of Infinity of existence, our evolving consciousness; thus humanity is ultimately floating in, trusting in, the spirit, energy, and grace of Cosmic Love (Watson & Smith, 2002). It is this Infinite field of Love, as cosmic energy, which envelops us, also becomes a universal field to which we all belong and to which we have access for healing self and Other. It is that which we resort to, are required to surrender to, when we are most alone, despairing, suffering, longing, and hurting; at the same time, most grateful for when we experience joy, hope, and healing insights that come after or during the midst of pain and darkness.

13

Love and the Heart's Code

Emerging Field of Cardio-Energetics and Heart-Centered Living

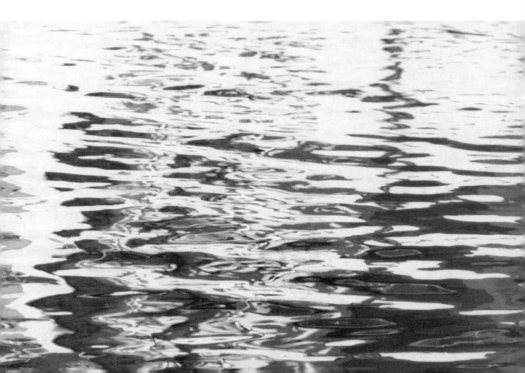

When you awake, your heart is an expression of Spirit, an expression of Love, expression of Life. Miracles happen all the time, because those miracles are performed by the heart. The heart is in direct communication with the human soul, and when the heart speaks . . . something inside you changes; your heart opens another heart and true love is possible.

Don Miguel Ruiz (1999). *The Mastery of Love*, p. 190

Recent developments in mind-body medicine are discovering new connections between the intelligence, sounds, and energy of the heart, referred to "cardio-energetics" and L-energy (Life or Love energy) (Pearsall, 1998). This shift toward honoring a heart-centered evolution for humans is in stark contrast to our head-centered orientation to life.

The works of Pearsall (1998) and others are bringing to our attention clinical observations, empirical science, personal stories, and case studies to demonstrate that the heart stores energy and information that comprises the essence of who we are, suggesting an invisible *heart code.*

The central thesis of this thinking in cardio-energetics, is that "the heart and not the brain is where our most basic thoughts, feelings, fears, and dreams are gently but profoundly mediated, is becoming increasingly supported..." (Pearsall, 1998, p. 68). With this central thesis, he invites us to consider the recent findings from research in the field of neurocardiology, the study of the heart as a neurological, endocrine, and immune organ (Pearsall, 1998, pp. 68–69):

❀ "Neurotransmitters found in the brain have also been identified in the heart, establishing a direct neurochemical and electrochemical communication between the heart and the brain beyond purely neurological connections known to exist";

❀ The heart, through hormones, neurotransmitter, and what scientists call subtle quantum energies and Pearsall calls "L" info-energy (I am suggesting "L" = Cosmic Love), exerts at least as much control over the brain as the brain exerts over the heart;

❀ Drs. John and Beatrice Lacey of the National Institute of Mental Health report that there is direct evidence that the heart neurohormonally calls for a constant environmental update from the brain in order to organize the body;

❀ When the muscular walls of the heart's atria contract, the heart produces a hormone that profoundly affects every major organ of the body, including the brain. Called atrial naturetic factor (ANF), sometimes called peptide, this neurohormone communicates not only with the brain but directly with the immune system, the hypothalamus (which helps mediate our emotional state), and the pineal gland (which regulates the production of melatonin that is related to our sleep/wake cycle, again processes, and general energy level). The ANF from the heart also influences the thalamus and pituitary gland in the limbic or emotional part of our brain, an important center of our memory, learning, and emotions.

In addition to these findings, Pearsall further indicates that continuing neurocardiology research points toward the central role of the heart in our consciousness. This becomes much more than metaphor and is moving close to the complexity of revealing a "conscious heart," which our brain cannot yet imagine (p. 69).

The heart is unlike any other organ in the body, whereby we can hear, feel, and sense the workings of the heart. "It constantly oscillates with the information we need to live and to love. It communicates its info-energy to every cell in our body and other bodies . . . it provides a resonating reminder that we are sending and receiving the information of our soul" (Pearsall, 1998, p. 69).

Just as Teilhard de Chardin considers Love a form of unitive energy that brings all of life together, Pearsall too reminds us that energy of the heart (Love energy from the heart), referencing surgeon Sherwin Nuland (Pearsall, 1998, p. 41), is what keeps a human being in one piece. His cardio-energetic hypothesis suggests a Fifth force, which is associated with the identity of the human soul, reflecting a specific, yet subtle, energy, which is "vital" to our life force. Pearsall notes what James Hillman referred to as a "calling from within," a guiding force and a knowing in our "heart of hearts" what we are here to do and why we came here in the first place.

This view is not too unlike Florence Nightingale's insights whereby she was very clear that nursing (and maybe we now need to add *all healing* work) was/is a "spiritual calling"; and she asked us: "What are your *musts?* What is it you *must* do?" This is consistent with one of the messages of this book: Can we *remember* why we came? I believe, at some basic level, we came to this earth-plane to learn to Love, to Become, Be Love; at least that is my quest and insight for my existence and my *remembering*. This work comes from the heart, not the head, though, a major shift and shock to the brain and the ego.

In more straightforward language, others have suggested that four chambers of the heart carry four major forms of energy: Unconditional Love; Compassion; Harmony; Healing Presence (Day, 2003). In this frame of reference, one of our quests is to see the divine essence in everyone, practicing unconditional love as we live from the heart center in our daily world and work. In doing so, in her thinking, we create a circle of heart radiance, enbeautiment, true connection, communion, united in compassion, whereby joy, love, and inner peace are released.

In doing so, this is one way to work with both *Caritas* and *Communitas,* ever widening the concentric circles of caring consciousness and connections. In working from the radiance of the heart in this way, we are attuning to universal Love. When we shift from fear or head to heart and begin to repattern our lives/energy fields, it affects our entire life holographically. Further, as people change at the individual level, they see others differently, as teachers, or loving helpers, not as adversaries, enemies, or competitors. We move from Caritas to Communitas in this work, because what we are holographically communicating with the entire self, we likewise are contributing holographically to collective consciousness of humanity, affecting the universal field of infinity. It is in this way that we co-evolve with the universe in both Whitehead and Chardin views.

This shift suggests we are more able to manifest our intentions, re-patterning old ways of living, responding. Once one has shifted into this heart-centered living and experienced a re-patterning of one's field, it is not realistic to go back to previous patterns. Once attuned with the heart center, if we are not living from that space, we detect it more quickly. We recognize when we are responding from fear and shift quickly back to the heart center to self-correct. So what was a choice in the beginning now becomes essential to sustain our inner love, peace, caring. It is posited that to truly engage in healing work, one has to work from the heart center. Indeed, to be more specific, it is proposed that if we are serious about caring-healing practices, and as we wake up to this deeper reality of existence and love as the highest level of consciousness, practitioners of caring-healing will be/become radiating centers of love and light offering their presence in the moment, working from the heart center; whereby, they become conduits for connecting with Cosmic universal, infinite Love and are likewise contributing holographically to an evolving universe, moving more closely to Chardin's *Omega Point,* Levinas' *Originary Infinity of Love,* and Whitehead's *Causal Future/Eternal Now,* in which we are co-participants.

Along these same ancient lines of archetypal thought about the heart and its energetic field, Pearsall reported the alleged story of Michelangelo, where he "saw an image radiating from the heart of the person he was sculpting" (Pearsall, 1998, p. 42), suggesting the *fifth force* in this field. This *fifth force,* so to speak, is not only related to modern scientific thought but to ancient as well as contemporary views of the energy of the soul: the immaterial essence, the subtle yet vital force of life (Pearsall, 1998, p. 42). This subtle energy or vital *fifth force* emanating from the heart is now being connected with contemporary views in quantum physics (e.g., quarks, stars, waves, and particles) as well as notions of non-local energy consciousness that energetically connects the universe, and connects humans "at a distance," through such practices as love, caring, prayers, healing thoughts, distant healing, and so forth. This new insight is positing that there is an energetic intelligence from the heart (Infinity of Cosmic Love?), which has rules of its own and which operates by timeless connections, beyond time and space and temporality, as we have been conditioned to think in our mechanical models of the universe.

Pearsall raises the question about our ways of schooling ourselves and our institutions' fixation on the use of the mind, the head, the brain, and the cognitive rationality of thought. But what if we were required to cultivate and use the energy of the heart? Might we cultivate a more loving, caring, evolved humanity, remembering that Love is the highest level of consciousness?

Not only is the heart emerging as the energetic center for essence of the person, but it is also increasingly viewed as the center for connecting with others, loved ones and those in our midst. As Pearsall puts it, *"The brain may contain more cellular connections than there are in the stars in the Milky Way, but it is nowhere near as energetic as the heart. By bioscience's own measurements, the heart is five thousand times more electromagnetically powerful than the brain"* (Pearsall, 1998, p. 65).

MAKING CONTACT WITH OUR HEART

One of the other astonishing aspects of this growing field of cardio-energetics and concern for heart-felt orientation to living and healing is the concept of "cardio-contemplation"—an orientation I prefer to think of as "Heart-Deep Love contemplation"—nevertheless, the notion is that this mindfulness of focus on the heart is a form of meditation, but unique in that it focuses on the heart and loving-kindness and great Cosmic Love, filling one's heart center. It has been suggested this might be one way to connect with the notion of collective unconscious, on some subtle energetic level, that may be non-locally stored in the memory system of every cell of own body. Indeed, it is suggested by Pearsall that this may be a process that allows us to make contact with our soul, by tapping into our spiritual energy (Pearsall, 1998, p. 153).

This contemplative process of meditating on the heart and Cosmic Love emanating from its center may be a way to silently pause to vibrate with all the energy, feelings, and sensations of the moment, described as "amplified peace" (Institute of Heartmath, cited in Pearsall, p. 154).

This experience of implied peace in midst of pauses and silence is related to what T.S. Eliot called the "still point" in the dance of life.

> "... at the still point, there the dance is,
> But neither arrest nor movement. And do not call it fixity,
> Where past and future are gathered.
> Neither movement from nor towards,
> Neither ascent nor decline. Except for the still point,
> There would be no dance, and there is only the dance.
> T.S. Eliot, 1944, p. 15

This notion of still point, silently vibrating with heart and breath, is allowing "our heart to be open to its natural resonation with all the energies of the present moment and thereby expanding, freezing, or spiritually pausing to allow one's self to be completely immersed (present) in the present moment" (Rechtschaffen, in Pearsall, 1998, p. 154). This is congruent with Whitehead's notion of the eternal now, in a given moment, whereby past, present, and future become one; in the "caring moment," which transcends the usual felt sensation of physical-temporality of time and space whereby the "still point" is there in the middle of the dance of life. This space of amplified peace, still point, the space between the breaths, the void, is both full and empty—a space and place that are transcendent yet fully there. Athletes refer to this sensation as being in the zone; others as altered sensory perception, altered consciousness, and so forth. In other words, one has moved out of one's head and transcended the usual ego identity, allowing the heart and other sensations to be experienced.

Out of this increasing awareness of heart-centered practices, others are beginning to explore more explicitly how we can make contact with other hearts through heart-centered practices, or in "letting our hearts pray," to refer to Hawaiian practices reported by Pearsall (1998), as a way to uniting hearts at the energetic level.

Again, Pearsall reports that recent heart-to-heart info-energetic connection is not just a theoretical concept. Research shows that one person's heartbeat can be measured in another person by comparing electrocardiograms. This impact of heart energy connection according to Pearsall seems most measurable and noticeable when we are closer together, particularly when we physically touch, hold hands, and so forth; we facilitate "the polarity of the connection by holding right hand to left . . . we are creating an 'L' energy loop" (Pearsall, 1998, p. 164).

This phenomenon seems to relate to prayer in that it can be envisioned as Love, a merging of info-cardio-energy from one person to another, in the non-local sense. This thinking is beyond "sending energy" in the usual way it has been suggested through some models of energy and distant healing (including some of my earlier thinking in my book *Postmodern Nursing and Beyond*, Watson, 1999b). In this emerging model, energy does not go anywhere at all in the usual sense, but is everywhere always present, like a "fifth force," according to Pearsall (1998). We are not just influenced and being participants with this energy, but we are part of it. So, prayer, like meditation, and other transcendent experiences can be seen as a merging with this energy, or in "flow" (Csikszentmihalyi, 1990) with it.

Pearsall reports a growing hypothesis researched by Russek and Schwartz (in Pearsall, 1998, p. 169), which suggests that one person's heart seems to exchange energy with another's heart, and there is an exchange of energy between two people's hearts, acting somewhat like a tuning fork, resonating with both heart and brain one person to another.

Pearsall goes on to make the analogy that the heart may indeed be the soul's tuning fork, expressing the soul's code with every beat. In a group, there may be a resonating among the whole, if the people become focused and connected with the heart. In this sense, it is posited that cardio-energetics hypothesizes that the heart can serve as a magnetic pole, attracting heart/love energy. If one has an open, warm, loving heart, then "we allow God's infinite Love to happen to us. It is at these times when we are most loving and ready to receive another's heart" (Love) (Pearsall, 1998, p. 168). This relationship between heart, caring, love, and healing begins to merge.

In this context, a nursing leader in a hospital project in New York recently told me that the nursing staff was using my work on caring as a theoretical-philosophical foundation for their practice model. She confided in me that she wanted to develop a logo that said *"Caritas is Magnetic,"* in that they were using my concept of *Caritas and Love,* from my publications, as a means to transform nursing within, while also seeking status as a magnet hospital. I told her that the logo was appropriate and meaningful for more reasons than one, mentioning to her some of this latest thinking in the field of cardio-energetics. Within this framework, the model of caring and love indeed serves as a magnetic field attracting more Love/heart-felt energy into the system and can become a framework for not only Caring Science but for caring-healing practices.

However, it is our brain and cognitive limitations that insist on a separation of our existence from anything that may be a greater source of sovereign control and wisdom and knowledge beyond anything we currently understand and that we can/must yield to eventually. It is when we open our heart that we are *reminded* how "to be" and that we indeed *Belong* to that which is greater than any one separate person. It seems that when our heart is open, energy pours in from other hearts, and energy from this non-local field does indeed guide and nurture us into loving heart-to-heart bonds (Pearsall, 1998).

Such thinking deviates from our demand on our self to *DO*. Rather, the heart connection asks for more of our *Being,* requiring an inner quiet; it serves as an invitation of receptivity, accepting and welcoming in the sense that Levinas refers to as a hospitality toward Other, and yielding of separatist ego and cognitive-control exclusivity, to a higher/deeper source of sovereign Being-Belonging to/with the infinity, and family of, life itself. It is through this awareness and maybe awakening of the human spirit toward evolution of Cosmic Love as the highest level of consciousness that is our human destiny; that is, if we are going to survive as humans and a civilization into this millennium. Or as I heard Larry Dossey put it, something to the effect, "this century will have to be one of spirituality or it won't be one at all" (Colorado talk, 1999). That is, if we are going to make it out of this century alive, we have to engage in a more evolved consciousness, connecting us with infinity of Spirit.

Another way of understanding the mystery of the heart and Cosmic Love is that it may be that it is through the heart that we connect with this infinity of energy/spirit/Love, which is the energetic field of the universe in which we all reside. It may be that it is through the heart that we tune into the depths and heights of both our inner Divinity/Soul and outer Divinity/Spirit, which is the great Creator, God of all, regardless by what names we may use to describe and connect/relate to this infinite Source of all of life. As Pearsall puts it," It is surrendering the self, transcending the brain's illusion of control, resonating with 'L' energy (which is) the way the created becomes One with the Creator" (Pearsall, 1998, p. 166).

Barbara Brennan's work affirms these hypotheses and more through her energy-light healing work. As she put it: "Everything we think, say, and do holographically affects everyone else through the life energy fields" (Brennan, 1993, p. 177). Thus, in this evolving consciousness context for Caring Science, we are energetically connected to all people in the world. In this sense, the heart is considered the bridge to Love and an evolving humanity. As we evolve in our considerations of science and practice alike, these emerging directions have enormous implications for our personal and professional future.

14

Holding Holy Space in Our Face, Hands, and Heart

A Caring Science perspective invites a new awakening, a new awareness of the sacredness of our work and our world. As Levinas indicated, he saw his work not just as ethics, but approaching the holy. That was his pursuit; I share that longing with him. When we delve into Mystery, Infinity, Energy, evolving Consciousness, and Spirit and begin to honor, as well as yield to, that which surrounds and contains the life field: Cosmic, Universal field of Love, as the unitive force of all of life, then we have to pause to bow down to the sacred nature of this caring-healing work and service of our life and being in the world. When we step into this great circle of Caring Science work, we step into sacred space, because we are touching the life force energy, the mystery of the inner soul's journey. We in turn are co-participants in this journey toward inner healing and unknowns and ambiguities and wonders that cannot be contained in conventional science cosmologies, traditions, nor worldview assumptions.

This thinking then moves us to new conceptualizations of the caring-healing practitioners and their very human presence, which becomes part of the healing process, or part of the disruption, depending upon our awakening. Once we relocate ourselves in a Caring Science framework, we are challenged, if not forced, to rethink the significance of the human practitioner and the nature of the consciousness, the authenticity of his/her heart-centered work.

Aspects of this shift toward considering the importance of the practitioners and their human consciousness, and presence, as part of the healing process have been addressed by Quinn (1992) in a classic paper. She conceptualized evolving perspectives of the nurse as one who holds "sacred space" as he/she becomes the environment, but rethinking what we mean by environment. In a Caring Science context, this thinking about the nurse moves to consider these ideas as relevant to any caring-healing practitioner.

Quinn acknowledged environment as a central focus for nursing (all healing practitioners); but environment was core to Florence Nightingale's paradigm for health. In reconsidering environment for Caring Science, Quinn's work is relevant. Drawing upon and modifying her views, we can identify at least three ways of conceptualizing the environment and the practitioner's place within the environmental field. (She identified two, but I am expanding these notions.)

First, by thinking of the environment as separate from the practitioner and client, and something you modify in the external world, but it is separate from serious consideration or attention with respect to the caring-healing process. It is confined to physical, external environment and is not considered a part of the process that is affecting either the practitioner or the client. In this consciousness, the practitioner may or may not attend to the environment, other than to view it and use it as a place of practice for the physical plane of work. In this framework, one considers whether the environment is tidy, clean, aesthetic, functional, and so forth, from a strictly external basis that is confined to personal taste, comfort, privacy, safety, environmental hazards, etc.

A second way of viewing the environment that Quinn identified is to think a step beyond just the environment being the site of practice in an external, physical sense, but to think of the practitioner and the client as *being* the environment together. In this view, practitioner and client are looking out from the same vantage point into the same environment. If one drew upon a theoretical-philosophical framework to understand this view of environment, in a Rogerian–Unitary Science scheme or Newman's Health as expanding consciousness scheme or a transpersonal Caring view, the practitioner would be concerned with *patterning the environmental field* (Quinn, 1992, p. 26). So, the practitioner and client pattern the environment to promote healing, harmony, comfort, a sense of well-being, aesthetic pleasure, and so forth.

In this second conception of environment, the questions we might ask are:

❋ What can the practitioner *do* to create (pattern) an environment that is more healing for the client?

❋ What could be deleted, and what could be added?

❋ What color, light, sound, activity, temperature, and so forth, could be addressed?

These dimensions of environment are, in essence, many of the issues with which Nightingale was concerned (Quinn, 1992, p. 27) but also now converge with contemporary unitary science theories of the evolving human and caring-healing and health. After appraisal and alteration of the environment in this second level of awareness, the practitioner, *being in* the environment, would then turn attention to the use of particular caring-healing modalities to assist in patterning a more healing environment. Modalities such as imagery, visualization, relaxation, music-sound, art, and so forth, might be "used to alter the environment with which the client is interacting at that moment such that a more harmonious healing process is possible" (Quinn, 1992, p. 27). While this conception of the environment is an evolved level beyond paying no conscious, intentional attention to the environment, and while this view is theoretically grounded in that the practitioner is viewed as integral with the client's environment, the practitioner, nevertheless, continues to act from the position of a separate self *in* the environment; shaping and sculpting it are efforts to facilitate client healing (Quinn, 1992, p. 27).

Now, if we take another leap of consciousness related to the place of the practitioner in the environmental field, consistent with an evolving Caring Science awareness, we have another view. In this evolving perspective, described by Quinn (1992, and modified here), in addition to acknowledging the environment as a functional, physical place for practice (first view) and in addition to thinking of the practitioner as *in* the environment, (second view described by Quinn), she and I now invite us to *consider the practitioner and their evolved caring consciousness, presence, intentionality, heart-centered foci, and so forth, as the environment!* Now, this evolved view of human practitioner *as the environment* has powerful implications for the evolved consciousness of the practitioner. To paraphrase Quinn (p. 27): In this perspective, the practitioner turns toward her or his understanding of the *practitioner-self* as an energetic, vibrational field, integral with the client. This view is related to heart-centered practices described above, acknowledging not only unitary views of science, but new views of the significance of practices that flow from a higher level of consciousness of caring-love, connecting with the infinity of energy/universal love/spirit, connecting spirit-to-spirit in the unitary field.

Questions posed by Quinn and adapted for this evolved conceptualization of environment might be:

❋ If *I am the environment,* how can I *be* a more caring-healing environment?

❋ How can I *become* a safe space, a sacred vessel, a holy space for this client and his/her soul's inner healing journey?

❋ In what ways can I look at, into this person (how am I to *face this Other*) to draw out healing? Wholeness that is already present?

❋ How can my heart-centered presence and loving/caring consciousness help to align in this moment with energy/infinity of Spirit/Universal love?

❋ How can I use my heart-centered awareness, my consciousness, my *Being,* my presence, my voice, my touch, *my face, my hands* for healing?

To relate this evolving view of the practitioner *as* the environment, now we can go back to the extant caring theories and the findings reported by Smith (1999). Perhaps for new reasons, we can see that in the practitioner-client field is one entity, connecting with infinity of universal field of energy/spirit/love, and perhaps we can better grasp that:

❋ Caring is a way of manifesting intentions;

❋ Caring is a way of appreciating (and participating in pattern);

❋ Caring is a way of attuning to dynamic flow (in the moment, in the universal field);

❋ Caring is a way of experiencing the Infinite (by working from heart-center and working toward one's own evolving consciousness, becoming more and more aware of the presence of infinity Love/spirit/universal energy);

❋ Caring is a way of inviting creative emergence (by practitioner holding sacred/holy space through intentional use of heart energetics, consciousness of caring and love, whereby the mystery, infinity can enter into the now).

In this way of considering the evolved human practitioner, we can literally become the healing environment. On another level of understanding this view, Quinn (1992) uses therapeutic touch as exemplar of practitioner consciousness *as* environment in that its modus operandi is a shift in the consciousness of the practitioner, through which clinical experience and empirical study demonstrate that through this process of centering there can also be a shift of consciousness of the recipient. (Another interpretation within an exploratory Caring Science context, based upon Levinas and Logstrup, is that through centering, one is allowing oneself to empty out and become an instrument for cosmic love to flow through one; thus, one opens up to universal field of infinity, wider cosmology, essentially spiritual and energetic, immanent and transcendent.)

This thinking is based upon a given that we are interconnected to all of life through the universal infinity field. Our consciousness is not separate and apart but integral with all consciousness. We can knowingly participate in this web of interconnection/oneness toward re-patterning and healing ourselves and others (Quinn, 1992). Therapeutic touch as exemplar is thought of as a re-patterning of her or his own energy field in the direction of expanded consciousness; a consciousness experienced as unified, harmonious, peaceful, and so forth (Quinn, 1992, p. 29). Quinn goes on to use the metaphor of sound, suggesting the pattern, vibration of the nurse's higher energetic field of consciousness becomes a tuning fork, resonating at a healing (Love) frequency, in which the client attunes to, resonates, to that frequency.

This view of Quinn's 1992 work now takes on new meaning in light of the new theories, hypotheses, and research in the field of cardio-energetics and heart-centered resonancy from one person to another. To repeat previous comments, then we see again that the model of caring and love indeed serves as a magnetic field attracting more Love/heart-felt energy into the system and can become a framework for not only Caring Science but for caring-healing practices.

In our caring-healing practices, we see again, both from this conceptualization as well as new theories and research, when we open our heart that we are *reminded* how "to be" and that we indeed *Belong* to that which is greater than any one separate person. It seems that when our heart is open, energy pours in from other hearts, and energy from this non-local field does indeed guide and nurture us into loving heart-to-heart bonds (Pearsall, 1998).

To evolve in our humanity and our science, we "are called to look anew at how we knowingly participate in our interconnected unitary universe. We can no longer view the environment, nor the practitioner as being 'out there'" (Quinn, 1992). We *Belong* and *Become* the environment for our clients, colleagues, communities, systems, world, and ourselves. So, in entering into this new conceptualization, theorization, actualization, we enter into and hold holy and sacred space for all whom we encounter and touch. In doing so, we are healed. And once again we are reminded, and *remember* once again, our most authentic human service. This caring-healing work then becomes one of the greatest gifts we can offer to Other, to humanity and to self. In the process, we transcend our limited professional orientations and ourselves. Together, all who enter into this perspective of Caring Science unite and co-evolve together in our expanding universe. Together we co-create a new reality for sharing our awakening to a higher consciousness. Our movement toward universal Love in turn manifests in our daily work and life. But this process is not without some personal awakening, re-patterning of consciousness toward this higher unitary field of universal Caring/Love.

15

From "Facing Our Humanity" to "Faces of Water"

Artistic Reflections Revealing How Different States of Consciousness Affect Our World

This section uses art and metaphor to capture the relationship between our consciousness, our thoughts, and how they are manifest in our environmental field through water crystals. Metaphorically, if the majority of the human body consists of water, it is interesting to ponder the relationship as to how our thoughts are reflected in our body, our life, and our world.

Recent work of Masaru Emoto (2002) from Japan has captured creative and scientific, if not environmental, attention regarding the role of water in our life and our world. His research of various kinds of water, such as water in a human body, water in daily life, and water on the Earth, reveals new knowledge and insights, not just about scientific aspects but from the personal. For example, his work indicates that water is a mirror reflecting our mind.

In this section of the book, and through this recent Japanese work, we metaphorically, ethically, scientifically, and personally can see for new reasons:

In Facing Self—Facing Other:
We now see that our
Consciousness of Love/Caring or Non-Caring
Is manifest in *Faces of Water.*

Emoto's research and high-powered photography, using Magnetic Resonance Analyzer and micro-cluster, help us capture the mysteriousness of water and how it reflects back on our humanity and evolving consciousness—vividly revealing the unity of our human-environment field.

More specifically, this work and photography demonstrate how our thoughts, our music, our ecology affects the crystalline formation of water, revealing messages about our self we need to heed. This art world of Japanese photography shows us how different forms of Consciousness change the composition of Water visually and microscopically. It signifies subtle energy changes that are reflected in frozen water crystals, revealing how different states of consciousness affect the anatomical structure of water.

BACKGROUND: WATER, HUMANS, AND EARTH

Emoto (2002, p. 8) reminded us that water accounts for about 95% of the fertilized egg when the ovum of the mother and sperm of the father meet each other and become a fertilized egg. The amount of water in a matured human body is 70%, and we live surrounded by water every day until we die. Indeed, we are reminded that Water is the source of all of life. This Planet Earth is called the "Water Planet," with about 70% of its surface covered with water, similar to human body (Emoto, 2002, p. 8). Pursuing the mystery and intrigue of water led

Emoto to develop a method of freezing water crystals and then photographing the crystals, revealing the beauty and wonder of each crystal. Some were lovely, others were ugly. The water crystals form a solid substance, with orderly configured atoms and molecules; through his unique process of freezing the different water crystals at 5° C below 0, Emoto was able to photograph samples; he and his organization and colleagues have now photographed and stored about 10,000 pictures in 4½ years (Emoto, 2002, p. 15). What is being uncovered in this remarkable work is the "message from water" about our life and consciousness.

What Emoto reports is that, through this work, he came to understand that by observing the water crystalline structures, through basic criteria of whether they were beautiful or not by just observation, they felt the water was basically trying to express itself, even when not beautiful. In other words, he understood these crystal pictures show different "faces of water," and even if water is not pure and clear, it expresses through the crystal that it "wants to be clear water, and is trying hard to become clear water" (p. 18).

Emoto's work spans many areas of photography and research, including Japanese and U.S. drinking water, water from clear sources in mountain lakes and streams, as well as water from polluted sources, revealing the different *faces of water*. What is most germane to this text is how water crystals reveal different faces according to their nature or source or the nature of the consciousness, which has affected the water. For example, one aspect of his book, *Messages from Water*, is his presentation of the story of ever-changing water; how water is affected by sound of music, both positively and negatively. Likewise, he reveals graphically how different messages to water such as "you make me sick" or "love/appreciation" are manifest in the crystalline structure of the water; in addition, his artistic work reveals how "showing a person's name to water," e.g., Adolph Hitler or Mother Teresa, reveal how water expresses itself differently. In other words, he goes on to demonstrate how water reflects people's consciousness and how water is changed by people's consciousness. Whether one wishes to consider this work artistically, metaphorically, scientifically, or literally, the messages from water are profound reminders of our unity and our consciousness connection with our world. We are our environment; the human-environment is *one* field, and our positive and/or negative approaches to life are revealed in the very structure of our consciousness and environment, our world.

These images have profound implications if we consider we are more than half water. We are left to ponder how our consciousness is affecting our inner life and those of others in our field, both near and non-locally. This remarkable art and science of water awaken us to a new consciousness and a new beauty that allows us to participate in unfolding the beauty and love in our inner and outer world. We are creating our human-environmental field, for better or for worse; we are creating beauty/appreciation/love or non-beauty; we are participants through our own field of consciousness, either allowing beauty to express as natural order or contributing to nature's distortion.

But the fact remains that *we hold beauty/natural order/life in our hands;* it is through *faces of water* that we can see, perhaps more clearly, the themes in this book: Through Levinas' notion of *Facing Self–Facing Other,* mirrored through *Faces of Water,* we can see Logstrup's reality that we quite literally *Hold our Human and Environmental World in Our Hands.* A Caring Science seeks to honor and participate in this unfolding universe in a way that unfolds the Love and beauty that is already there, waiting to express itself, with and through us, by entering into the heart-centered, divine dance with Infinity itself. The following photographs capture the different messages from *Messages from Water* (Masaru Emoto & (C) I.H.M. Co., Ltd):

> *Commentary:* "This is one of Beethoven's most famous symphonies and is a bright, fresh and joyous piece. This beautiful crystal supports the fact that good music positively affects water."

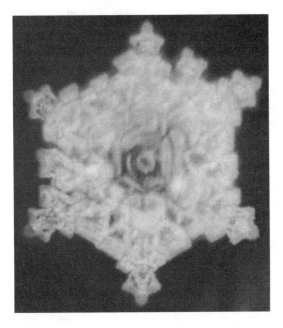

❊ **Figure 15-1** Water crystals from Beethoven's "Pastorale."

Commentary: "This symphony is a soulful song that seems to pursue beauty the most of any of the works of Mozart. A piece of deep thought that seems almost like a prayer to beauty. This music quietly heals the heart of its listeners. This crystal is so beautiful and graceful that it's as if it's speaking on behalf of the composer's feelings."

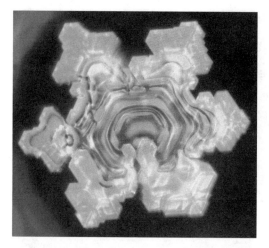

❉ **Figure 15-2** Water crystals from Mozart's "Symphony no. 40 in G Minor."

Commentary: "Through this famous violin piece, the crystal seems as if it has been enchanted by the sound of the music. The branches of the water crystal stretch out freely. This picture gives the impression that the crystal is dancing merrily."

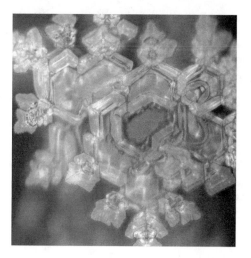

❉ **Figure 15-3** Water crystals from Bach's "Air for the G String."

Commentary: "This is a picture of crystal of water that formed after being exposed to a CD of music from the sound track of the 'Seven Years in Tibet.' We were able to take a picture of a powerful and beautiful crystal. We can reaffirm the ancient knowledge that the Sutra talks to people's souls and has a strong and positive energy that can heal people's feelings."

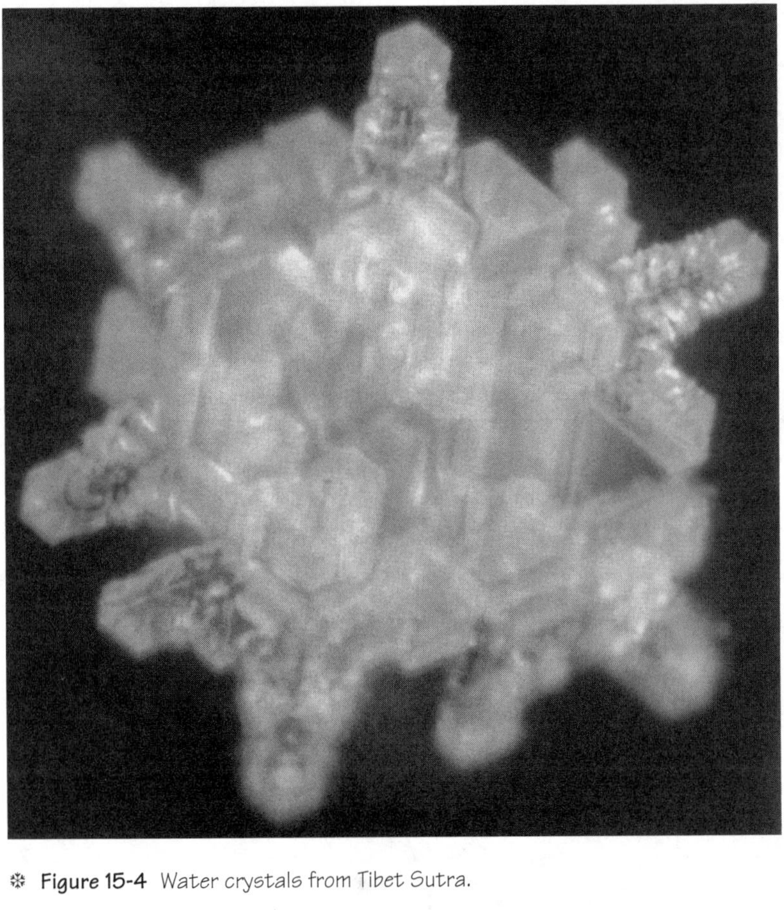

❄ **Figure 15-4** Water crystals from Tibet Sutra.

Commentary: "This music is filled with anger and seems to be denouncing the world. Subsequently, this crystal's basic well-formed hexagonal structure has broken into perfect pieces. The water seems to have reacted negatively to this music. We are not saying that heavy metal music is bad, only that there must have been a problem with the lyrics. This is merely an example."

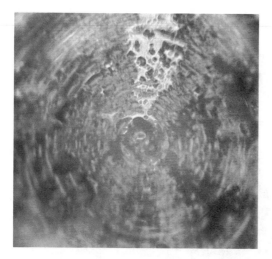

❄ **Figure 15-5** Water crystals from heavy metal music.

Commentary: "People's consciousness contained in love and appreciation. We took pictures of numerous crystals from this sample but this was the very first beautiful crystal we saw. Indeed, there is nothing more important than love and gratitude in this world. Just by expressing love and gratitude, the water around us and in our bodies changes so beautifully. We want to apply this in our daily lives, don't we? Strong resemblance to the crystal and the words 'Thank you' in another photo was a happy coincidence."

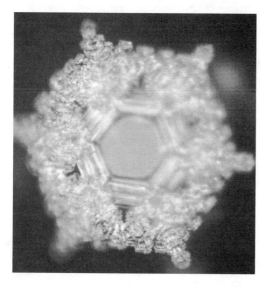

❄ **Figure 15-6** Water crystals shown Love/Appreciation.

Commentary: "What do you think?"

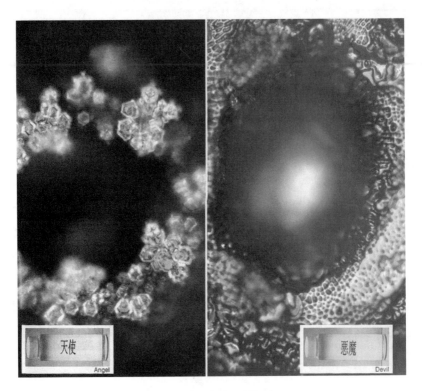

❖ **Figure 15-7** Water crystals shown Angel and Devil.

Commentary: "On January 17, 1995, the Great Hanshin-Awaji Earthquake occurred in Kobe. Three days afterwards we took pictures of the crystals found in the tap water in Kobe, that was available at the time. It is as if the water captured the fear, panic, and deep sorrow of the people immediately after the earthquake. The crystals were completely destroyed. It was a picture that made people shudder. We felt that we could not make this public because of the horror of its extreme misery. However, 3 months after that . . . Helping hands and sympathy from all over the world were given to the people of Kobe. Also since no riots occurred many people praised the people of Kobe. Although the rubble piled up high, people were able to restore their environment due to the kindness and warmth of others. This crystal seems to have collected those feelings also."

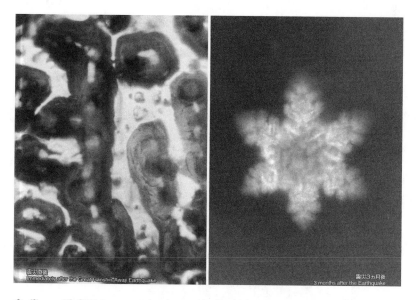

❊ **Figure 15-8** Water crystals changed by People's Consciousness: Water after Great Earthquake in Kobe, Japan, 1995.

16

Metaphysical-Ontological Mandala for a Caring Science Wheel of Knowledge

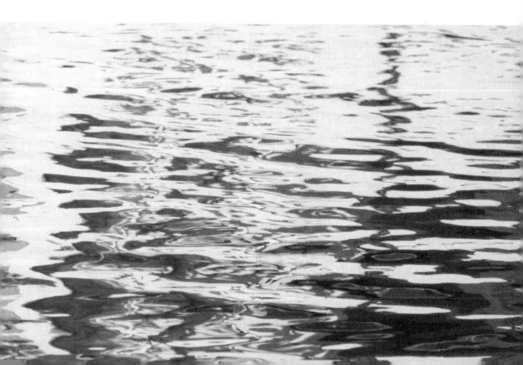

As we engage in Caring Science, we are directed toward a level of depth in trying to understand multiple ways of knowing and Being-Becoming, an approach that attempts to integrate and include matter, body, soul, and Spirit (Wilber, 1998, p. 102). In this overall framework, there is no closure, no definite answers or final version of science or Caring or Caring Science per se; however, this work seeks to point toward a Caring Science that attempts to integrate/reintegrate the observer with the observed, subtle matter and dense matter—the imma-nent with the transcendent-transpersonal. Thus, ancient wisdom tradi-tions, beliefs, and archetypal lines of knowing with contemporary science unfold in such a way that we are honoring the evolution of human consciousness—moving the human closer toward the Infinite Source of universal Love, which surrounds, contains, and holds all. In a Caring Science model, we seek new conceptualizations; frameworks for accom-modating the relationship and intersection between and among moral, metaphysical, ontological, and epistemological considerations as a means to knowledge development, forms of inquiry, practices, and living.

In addition to the Levinas' and Logstrup's philosophical and moral starting point for Caring Science, Wilber's Integral approach to a reconstructive science, in spite of his rejection of anything metaphys-ical, still, with some modification, probably comes as close to an orienting empirical framework for Caring Science as anything that currently exists. Thus, his work helps to relocate Levinas and Logstrup within both a conventional and contemporary Caring Science context (Wilber, 1998, p. 103). (See Table 16-1, based upon Wilber's 4-quadrant

Table 16-1

Mandala's Medicine Wheel Model Knowledge Based Upon Wilber's Four-Quadrant Model

INTERIOR	EXTERIOR
Subjective: inner experiential world Personal meaning; phenomenological view **"I" Knowledge**	Objective: external world **"IT" Knowledge**
INTERSUBJECTIVE	INTEROBJECTIVE
Collective: social meanings, culture, norms Ethnographic views **"WE" Knowledge**	Social-community outcomes **"IT" Knowledge**

model.) Wilber's multiple perspectives scheme allows subjectivity-objectivity, matter-spirit, to be incorporated into both the individual and collective levels of analysis. In this scheme, any phenomena can be examined from at least four dimensions: inside, outside, individual, and collective forms. Also, the scheme has the potential to allow for an intersection between the empirical, the ontological-ethical phenomena such as consciousness, caring-healing relationship: it incorporates the "I," the "It," and the "We." Thus, Wilber's scheme provides us with four dimensions of each level of existence, each phenomenon of interest.

Questions related to the impact of the caring-healing relationship on observable, measurable outcomes are upper right quadrant questions; questions related to how the relationship is manifest in and impacts on collections of individuals and systems of health care are lower right quadrant questions.

Upper and lower Right External outer world foci in Wilber's model accommodate the current interest in evidence-based practices; that is, empirically focused research and outcomes that focus on external criteria at either the individual or group level. As already noted above, with attention to the Left side of the model, we realize that the external focus alone is inadequate and insufficient to ensure a Caring Science perspective of human phenomena at either the individual or societal level. Likewise, a focus on the left side alone is equally inadequate. Wilber acknowledges each area is important, yet partial.

As pointed out in the State of the Art section of this book, which captures the disciplinary views and research of caring within nursing, make us increasingly aware of the importance of the Upper and Lower Left quadrant concerns. It is the Upper and Lower Left foci that incorporate individual, family, and community with culture, meaning, symbolism, rituals, metaphors, archetypal images, and influences affecting one's health and illness experiences.

Wilber's model is highly congruent with contemporary nursing grand theories and caring theories. For example, Martha Rogers, Margaret Newman, Paterson and Zderad, and Parse and Watson would point toward unitary perspectives as well as the Upper Left Quadrant; Leininger's transcultural care theory would accommodate both Lower Left and Right Quadrants (Fiandt, Forman, Megel, Pakieser, & Buirge, 2003).

Each of these perspectives from the four-quadrant model demonstrates that there are multiple and diverse ways of knowing, being, doing, responding, perceiving, thinking, and experiencing. All of these aspects affect our inquiring; this evolving, expanding view is not only necessary, it is required if we are to continue to pursue a more whole picture of our human caring-healing and health phenomena and human experiences out of the left-side phenomena of meanings and interpretations that affect external outcomes.

This model offers the ability to see parts and whole; the self as an individual and as a member of family-group-community. Further, it can serve as a values lens to see what we are overlooking, as well as where some extant knowledge can be located within the big picture, revealing at microscopic as well as macroscopic level (Fiandt, Forman, Megel, Pakieser, & Buirge, 2003, p. 135).

In addition to the left-right/upper-lower questions and locations of phenomena for inquiry, Caring Science also acknowledges that any caring-healing relationship is a process and phenomena that involves individuals, intersubjectivity, and relationships, and meanings at all levels. Knowing and knowledge involve a mutual, simultaneous process whereby there is the possibility of opening to the Infinity of Universal field of Love that surrounds and enfolds the entire Integral model of science. Caring Science honors the Universal field that comes before Being, surrounds all.

The Integral model of Knowledge indicates that those interested in changing, growing, and evolving in their methods of inquiry can use this multiple lens as a guide and pathway toward accommodating expanded views of knowledge and knowing and the epistemological-ontological-metaphysical evolutions necessary for Caring Science.

The Appendices included at the end of the text contain exemplars of the Caring Science model. The paper by Quinn, Smith, Ritenbaugh, Swanson, & Watson (2003) serves as a model for Caring Science inquiry related to caring-healing relationships. It identifies different forms of assessment and measurement tools, both standard and emergent, and novel ones, which are needed to encompass the full range of knowledge needed, consistent with the Wilber model and the search for all ways of knowing in Caring Science. One of the features of the Caring Science inquiry is to preserve the phenomena of relationship and unity, external and internal, microscopic and macro worldview to be present, while still creating novel forms for inquiry for different levels of analyses. Such efforts allow for all types and shapes of knowledge to be honored, systematically pursued, and located within a bigger picture of science.

A visual image of Wilber's Integral Model is modified and expanded to reflect a Caring Science orientation (Figure 16-1). It contains an overlay of the Medicine Wheel, or Mandala within the context of a circle. Instead of four quadrants, a circle, represented by the Medicine Wheel, can symbolize harmony and connection with a larger universe and natural elements of this universe: Earth, Air, Fire, Water and the sacred directions of the universe, conveying the connectedness of all. This broader view accommodates Levinas and Logstrup as well as Caring Theories and their notions of Infinity/Love and Universal field, beyond the empirical subjective-objective dialectic of knowledge

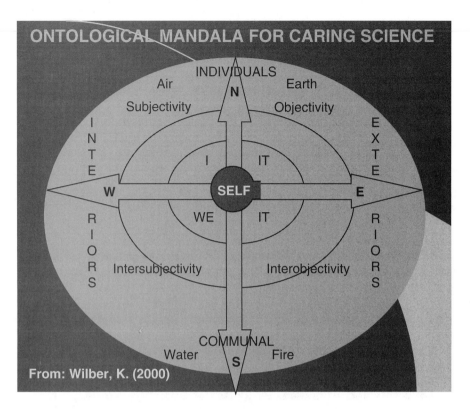

ONTOLOGICAL MANDALA FOR CARING SCIENCE

INDIVIDUALS

Air — N — Earth

Subjectivity — Objectivity

I — IT

W — SELF — E

WE — IT

Intersubjectivity — Interobjectivity

COMMUNAL

Water — S — Fire

INTERIORS

EXTERIORS

From: Wilber, K. (2000)

❖ **Figure 16-1.** Ontological mandala for Caring Science. Based on Ken Wilber's Original Knowledge Scheme, with Mandala/Medicine Wheel Overlay (Wilber, 1998. *The Essential Ken Wilber.* Boston: Shambhala, p. 103).

and humans. The human person is in the center, indicating that we stand in the sacred center of all, connecting with the web of life and all ways of knowing/being/doing for and with all elements of nature and all aspects of the Universe.

This expanded view of the Integral model with the Medicine Wheel/circular overlay reminds us that all things have spirit and life, including rivers, oceans, rocks, earth, air, fire, water, sky, plants, and animals. Within a Caring Science model, it is necessary to remind ourselves that we are spirit made whole; non-manifest to manifest field, connected to and Belonging to the Infinity of Cosmos and the Universe, before separating as individuals and other entities. The visual image of circle, embracing the four quadrants, reveals a transpersonal view of caring and humanity in that our being is both embodied yet transcendent.

The other dimension of this expanded model is that it makes more explicit that the human is the one who is determining the way we view knowledge and our world. The human is the one who uses self-reflexive consciousness and intentionality to co-create different worlds. Thus, our experience and views of knowing will be sacred or secular partly according to the purpose and intent we bring to it (Reason, 1993, p. 9). If we take a strict materialistic-utilitarian-separatist view of the planet as non-living matter, then that is the way our knowledge and our planet/earth will be (Reason, 1993). On the other hand, if we take a Caring Science Cosmology embracing Infinity of Love as Universal connection for our Belonging and Being-in-the-world, then we can see the self-other, planet and earth and cosmos as ensouled; then our views of life and knowing will unfold to us as living spirit (Reason, 1993, p. 9). To a large extent, it is a matter of our human intention, our evolving consciousness.

CARING SCIENCE MANDALA/MEDICINE WHEEL AS COSMOLOGY OF KNOWLEDGE/KNOWING

Our cosmological context becomes the social, political, cultural, and spiritual force that shapes the life of a person, community, and civilization (Baldwin, 1998, p. 21).

The context/cosmology of Caring Science represented by an expanded Integral model can become a collective image by which something is seen and understood differently (Baldwin, 1998); that is, the space within and around a circle shifts the context from ordinary to sacred. It also connects the harmonies of the universe, helping to bring about order of the whole (Fincher, 1991, p. 10).

Baldwin reminds us that a circle context is important, in that our context suggests how a culture changes. And context, such as a circle, mandala, or medicine wheel image of knowledge, prepares us to consider new ideas, a collective mind that is ancient and contemporary, making room for a deep well of knowing and communion between and among all things, our ancestral past, our present, and the future we are free to co-create. Thus, an even greater reason to consider Caring Science within the context/cosmology of a circle; this becomes worthy of our intention, our attention, as a way of embracing and envisioning our world and our science with a sacred lens toward all of life.

17

Re-Patterning Self for Caring-Healing

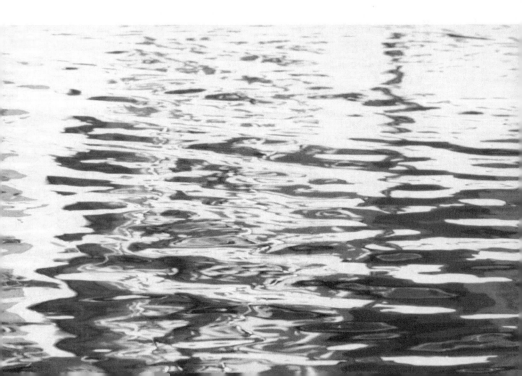

In addition to an explicit focus on Love, both human and Cosmic, as inherent evolving human consciousness for Caring–Healing work, and Caring Science, there are human self-care knowledge and practices that are necessary for us to honor for our re-patterning. This re-patterning is especially true if we are to engage in caring-healing work more fully and undertake the complexity of exploring human experiential phenomena for Caring Science.

Indeed, we see from earlier research related to caring relationships that, without an awakening and awareness of our very Being, our presence, intentionality, and consciousness AS *the field/environment,* we can actually be destructive to self and others. For example, the work of Halldorsdottir (1991) is again another reminder of the moral and practical importance of our caring presence/relationship in a given situation. For example, we know from this classic work that when there are so-called "professional caring relationships" that actually harm the client, this is largely due to the practitioner's often unconscious use of manipulation, coercion, abuse, humiliation, or other forms of physical, mental, emotional, or spiritual violence. This biocidic form of non-caring can be attributed to the practitioners' need for their own evolving and re-patterning from fear to love, from a lower level consciousness to a higher level; a shift perhaps from head-centered/personality/ego-centered work to heart-centered, higher consciousness movement. In her work, Halldorsdottir indicated that a "Type 1 biocidic relationship" involves the transfer of negative energy or darkness to the other (Halldorsdottir, 1991, p. 39). This is a stark contrast to the most evolved caring relationship, the Biogenic Type 5 Caring, which becomes life-giving. Thereby, the caring consciousness (cardio-energetic Love energy) energetically emanates a quality of positive, if not loving, energy that potentiates healing.

In these emerging frameworks, we are called to attend to our own evolving consciousness and self-care practices for our own healing and re-patterning toward Caring/Loving intentionality and consciousness for healing. These areas can be considered *human ontological-heart-centered developmental tasks,* in contrast with technological or exclusively head-oriented developments for our professional practices, our science, and our humankind. Attention to this reality of caring/non-caring relationships and their consequences for self and other becomes increasingly necessary to assist with our human evolution if we are going to sustain our humanity, if we are to co-participate in moving humanity closer to honoring and connecting with the Infinity field of universal Love, from which deep caring and healing comes.

These human ontological heart-centered self-healing phenomena and practice processes include at least the following:

❄ Forgiveness;

❄ Gratitude;

❄ Surrender; and

❄ Compassionate Human Service.

In considering these human evolutionary tasks we are invited to ask new questions such as: How are we to Be–Become to locate ourselves in a living Caring Science Model for our caring-healing practices in our work and our world?

ONTOLOGICAL-HEART-CENTERED TASKS

In this emerging work, we cannot stand outside of our self and practice from a detached bystander point of view, nor can we practice from distant theories. In a Caring Science practice of caring and healing, it invites a new and deeper meaning to the concept of professional *discipline* in that *self-discipline* for one's own spiritual growth and evolution of consciousness is a necessary requirement to sustain.

Healing work is fast becoming part of our science mandates as well as our practice domains. Society, in general, is now expecting new dimensions of personal growth from the practitioners; otherwise, the practices are not authentic, nor congruent, with the expectations of the public in this growing field. Thus, the practitioners of caring and healing require more personal work than ever before: because we practice who we are; we research who we are; we teach who we are; we live who we are. So our very Being-Becoming more human and humane is what is at stake in healing work. We emanate our presence and radiate from our heart center in a given caring moment. But our presence can be head-centered or heart-centered, or we can unite head and heart and actions to connect with the infinity of Love; otherwise we are left with *a totalizing/an objectifying* of self and other.

Forgiveness

It is repeatedly being claimed, if not known and proclaimed since Biblical times and before, if one is to truly heal, one has to learn how to forgive. Forgiveness of self and other seems to be a deep psychological, spiritual, if not physical-biological, task that is necessary to cleanse our psychic soul for evolving toward Love and Caring. It may be that forgiveness is necessary for healing even at the physical level. Forgiveness is not so much for the other person, although it becomes a reciprocal process, but primarily it becomes an essential task to relieve our own suffering.

It has been advised that we must forgive those whom we feel have hurt us, even if we think what occurred was unforgivable. Somewhere along the way we learned to be resentful, angry, and retaliatory toward others whom we felt harmed us in some way, but in harboring those feelings for others we hold those feelings against ourselves.

Non-forgiveness is not only toward our self or another person; it also may be toward any situation or condition—past, present, future—that our mind refuses to accept (Tolle, 1999, p. 100). Yet, to truly forgive, we learn to relinquish our grievance as we learn that it serves no purpose but self-imposed suffering and pain. Once we forgive, we open our self to the flow of live energy. And as Tolle (1999, p. 100) again reminds us: "The mind cannot forgive. Only *you* can."

Therefore, we discover that we forgive for our own cleansing and mental clearing, mental health. We also forgive because we feel compassion for others and, therefore, ourselves. Forgiveness is an act of self-love.

In Logstrup's view, on the other hand, forgiveness is perhaps one of those sovereign feelings of human expression that are given to us as supreme; but we are charged to *remember again*. As Ruiz reminds us: "Forgive others, and you will see miracles start to happen in your life" (1999, p. 174). To forgive others, however, we have to learn first to forgive ourselves. Just like love, to love others, we have to have self-love. These practices require re-learning at this point in our head-oriented life and word and work, but become essential to our evolving humanity and our individual and collective healing.

Indeed, forgiveness might be at the heart and root of freeing us for the unconditional flow of Love to enter our lives again, allowing us to return to the sovereignty of *Becoming-Being* the Love and light that we already are but have to rediscover/*remember* again. As Tolle put it:

> Forgiveness is a term that has been in use for 2,000 years, but most people have a very limited view of what it means. You cannot truly forgive yourself or others as long as you derive your sense of self from the past. Only through accessing the power of Now, which is your own power, can there be true forgiveness . . . and you realize that nothing you ever did or that was ever done to you could touch even in the slightest the radiant essence of who you are (Tolle, 1999, p. 191).

Wisdom traditions and healing scripts suggest we start practicing; working on, forgiveness, right now in our daily lives, if we are to release our essence of humanity, the radiant essence of who we truly are.

Ruiz (1999) and others suggest we begin by making a list of everyone you believe you need to *ask* for forgiveness. Then ask them for forgiveness; this can be silently, in a form of prayer, through your dreams, or in person. Making a list of all the people who you feel have hurt you and all those whom you need to forgive can follow this. This includes parents, siblings, children, spouse, lovers, friends, officials, colleagues, events, life circumstances that wounded you, and so on, even forgiving your God, who in some conditions we may feel has betrayed or abandoned us.

The only way to recover forgiveness is to practice it again and again, keeping it current in our lives as circumstances and events trigger old responses of retaliation, judgment, anger, resentfulness, and so on. Doing a self-check on forgiving self, allowing non-judgmental, equanimity, and loving-kindness to flow from our hearts and flood our consciousness is one step along the way. This involves a daily practice, if not a moment-by-moment mindfulness, for a more reflective, heart-centered life.

This process of self-forgiving; of asking for others' forgiveness, and of forgiving others all becomes an act of power, of self-acceptance, self-love, and healing. Without engaging in this basic sovereign human expressive act, there can be no true healing, no authentic love and flow of infinite universal energy into our hearts and lives.

Gratitude

It seems that another personal practice that can contribute to re-patterning our consciousness and contributing to our evolving toward a higher consciousness for healing is cultivation of giving gratitude for life and all its blessings, in the midst of pain, despair, turmoil, change, and unknowns. It seems that in bowing down to the magnificence and wonder and miracles that are among us that we begin to see the world in a new way. Sometimes, just a shift into giving thanks, without complaints for what is upon us in a given moment, is transforming in itself.

A prayer, mantra that my minister often uses is: "Father, Mother God, the only one, thank you! I have no complaints!" In allowing surrender and humble presence before the gift of life itself, even if it is not as we would have it be in the moment, is not only healing but also enlightening. In cultivating the practice of giving thanks and gratitude for all, we see/feel/experience the wonder and majesty of the world in a given moment and often time and experiences stand still and/or are transformed, altered in perception and felt experience. Tolle (1999) refers to the practice of *NOW*. And it seems that pausing to be still, to be present, to bow down and give thanks for all our blessings in the middle of felt chaos, is a great teacher and another route to universal Love, universal infinity of energy for healing. As such, we are engaging actively in re-patterning our consciousness, reconnecting us with our Source, and in doing so we are not only sustaining our own individual humanity, but humanity collectively. It seems that in practicing gratitude, we open our heart-center, allowing love and wonder and even more gratitude, energy, creativity, to flow through us and our experiences, perceptions, and life events.

In this practice of giving gratitude, we open ourselves to new energy and life force, releasing negative attachments, which prevent us from honoring, experiencing all of life as a blessing and a teacher, reminding us of why we came here, helping us to both *remember* and evolve toward higher consciousness, allowing greater access to/with the universe/universal Love.

Surrendering

With our conditioned head-centered, ego-controlled focus of our lives, one of the most difficult lessons for our self-healing and re-patterning of ways of Being in the world is the practice of *surrendering*. When we are so oriented toward control, domination, with a sense of rational knowing that we are responsible for making things happen, the concept of surrendering is foreign to us and our ego world of operation. Nevertheless, it often is only through surrendering, in letting go of ego-sense of control and our efforts to make something happen, that we witness new possibilities unfolding in front of us. When we fixate on making, or trying to make, every effort to fix something that is wrong and does not conform to the way we think things should be, we create more pain and suffering in our lives.

It is in and through such disappointments in our efforts that we ultimately realize that we are not in control. It is often during major life crises, illness, trauma, and accidents, or when things go wrong from the way we think they should be, that we learn this hard lesson. Surrender is about learning to turn things over, to let go of ego, to realize that ulti-mately life is bigger and more grand than anything we can imagine, let alone control. And even in the worst case scenario when everything seems out of our control, when things fall apart, we may learn the deepest lessons about surrendering.

Tolle (1999) writes about surrender as not only the letting go of mental-emotional resistance to what *is* but also when we do ultimately surrender; the process becomes a portal into the unmanifested field of possibilities (p. 111). The more we resist surrendering to that which is greater than self, the more the feelings of separation, the more inner resistance builds, and the more cut off we are from our self, other people, the world around us.

The experience of surrender is closely tied to acceptance. It is as if we have a habit toward judging and labeling our perceptions and experiences, rather than just allowing them to be as they are. It is this reactive pattern with life that ultimately has to be surrender, through the simple act of accepting, not fighting just *what is, rather than what we wish it to be.* Tolle (2003) points out how difficult it is to "internally stand in opposition to what *is*" (p. 63): "Doing one thing at a time is how a Zen Master captured the essence of Zen, which means to be totally into what you are doing, giving it your complete attention, which is considered surrendered action, thus, empowered action (Tolle, 2003, p. 66). Again, according to Tolle's wisdom, it is our acceptance of what *is* that takes us to a deeper level where we can accept the moment as it is, resulting in the feeling of a sense of spaciousness within that is deeply peaceful.

Such deep acceptance and, thus, surrender is no longer dependent on external conditions or on the internal conditions of our constantly changing thoughts and emotions; the background of peace remains within (Tolle, 2003). What happens when such acceptance and surrender become part of our consciousness? We realize that all is fleeting, nothing is permanent, and the world cannot give anything of lasting value. As Tolle put it, the miracle occurs when we no longer place an impossible demand on every situation, person, place, or event; then life becomes more harmonious, more peaceful. This view is not to deny what is with negative feelings, but occurs when we no longer ask "Why is this happening to me?" Ultimately then, we realize and discover that "acceptance of the unacceptable is the greatest source of grace in this world" (Tolle, 2003, p. 71). We have learned to bear the unbearable in our heart, mind, and actions, and this awareness, reality takes us to peace.

Compassionate Human Service–Engaged Caring Practices

I am only here to be truly helpful.
I am here to represent Him who sent me.
I do not have to worry about what to say or what to do,
because He Who sent me will direct me.
I am content to be wherever He wishes, knowing
He goes there with me.
I will be healed as I let Him teach me to heal.
Marianne Williamson, 1992

I slept and dreamt that life was joy.
I awoke and saw that life was service.
I acted and behold, service was joy.
Tagore

Within Buddhist philosophy there is the concept of "engaged Buddhism." In that philosophy, those who are serving others in their community are working to earn what is referred to as "performing merits," which is a term used by laypeople who offer their time and energy to help with temple work. But more important, as Thich Nhat Hanh (2003, p. 100) indicates, it is to perform merits in the world of suffering, not in the temple, in that in serving others in need is serving the Buddha. It is a path to joy.

One way to understand compassionate human service and a sense of engaged caring is knowing that when we go to bed at night our talents, gifts, skills, and abilities have been used in a way that served others and made a difference, no matter how small. At a deep level of awareness our life's work is about spreading love (Williamson, 1992).

It is in this sense that we surrender our self to a higher/deeper purpose to serve outside of our ego self, whereby we may be instruments through which caring is radiated from self to other, contributing to a healing in the midst of daily work life. With such a commitment to engaged caring, our life has some greater sense of purpose beyond our self, whereby our talents, gifts, and skills may be more fully actualized toward compassionate human and community service.

Any career can be used as a means of engaged caring in the world. Any job is a means to contribute to a bigger picture of service to humanity, being a Bodhisattva in training; that is, one who is committed to inspire and help to heal all sentient beings by renouncing ego-focused living and working. Such practitioners do not retire from the world; rather, they practice the extraordinary in the midst of ordinary life, following a more enlightened path than ego-directed living-working in the world.

When we are troubled about what we are to do with our life and work, we can ask for guidance, we can offer gratitude for the gifts we have that seek an outlet for meaningful service toward a better world. This is both a local and specific, as well as a global and universal, challenge that invites each of us to consider our place in the larger universe. It is in this practice and awareness that we are part of co-creating a moral community and moral world.

Thus, engaged caring in the world—through informed action, manifest as compassionate human service—is how we proliferate caring and peace in the world. Our engaged service on behalf of that which is greater than us serves the whole. This notion is not just Buddhist philosophy but is evident in any spiritual practices, Christianity and Eastern religions alike.

Wherever there is suffering, pain, violence, illness, and despair in the world, which are everywhere, there is an opportunity to practice engaged caring or carry out compassionate human service in any caring occasion. As we do that, we do it not as a separate individual but as someone who belongs to a great heritage and tradition with others, as a gift of self-service to their community of fellow human beings.

Thich Nhat Hanh (2003) reminds us that when we carry out such actions of caring and peace into our lives and world, we connect with our whole lineage of blood ancestors; we are part of a sea of humanity that allows us to be supported by all the teachers and practitioners who came before within this tradition of compassionate human service, which is ultimately a spiritual tradition and practice, regardless of religious order one may wish to honor.

It is in this way that we and our life and service continue beyond our individual lifetime. For every person we touch with compassionate caring action, we are influencing humankind, in that caring begets caring and is carried forth into the future by radiating actions into the universe.

To practice engaged caring through compassionate service, we become more mindful of our actions and work from an intentionality to be present to others during their vulnerability and needs. It does not require perfection; it involves being and becoming more human, more humane, more open, more willing to accept the positive and negative realities of humanity with loving-kindness and equanimity, without blame or condemnation but with an open heart that unites us human to human.

It is through service, in doing what is in front of us to do, we can discover a lot about ourselves. Service to other at whatever level always involves being-in-relation to something that is other than self (Vaughn, 1995, p. 287). However, authentic compassionate human service cannot be based on self-sacrifice because that type of service is detrimental to the one who is served as well as the one doing the service. When service becomes a burden, it ends in burnout, as many nurses and health practitioners well know. It is when we are able to be more mindful, more open and loving toward self that we are motivated more deeply to express our love, gratitude, compassion toward others outside our self. In this way, our heart is open to serve another from a motivation of spiritual maturity, whereby we take reciprocal action, becoming an integral part of whatever we do. Then service is a natural expression of who we are (Vaughn, 1995). As Vaughn, influenced by Rudolph Steiner, put it, "The ideal is not 'out there', but is realized by the deliberate loving effort of the individual. As the universal is realized in the particular, ethical individualism is considered a natural expression of a free spirit . . ." (Vaughn, 1995, p. 104). It is, thus, through our compassionate engaged caring that we radiate collective energy into the universe. This energy both transcends us and transports us with support and strength to know we are making a difference in the world, contributing to a global caring ethic, through simple, engaged acts of compassion and loving-kindness one to another, regardless of whether the acts are large or small, no matter where they may occur.

18

Personal Remembering

Practicing Personal
Forgiveness,
Gratitude,
Surrendering

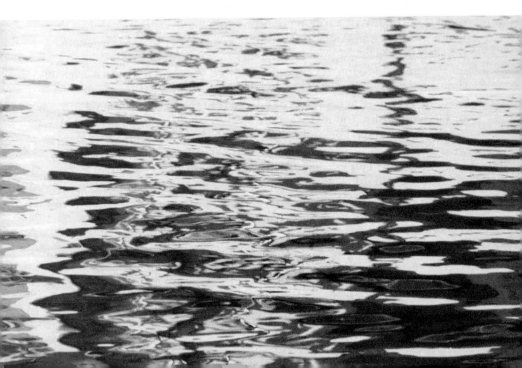

There are times in each of our lives in which powerful lessons and practices of forgiveness become more acute and mandatory for healing self, others, and a life situation. That has been the dramatic case for me in the past few years, due to major traumatic life changes from supposedly uncanny life situations.

As many who know me realize, in the late 1990s, I suffered a traumatic eye injury. The circumstances of the injury involved my 9-year-old grandson at the time. As a result, he and I now share a life-changing crisis that affected, and will affect, our lives forever. Some know this story, but to summarize for purposes here, I got in his line of fire, when he was swinging a golf club. Consequently I suffered long-standing pain, surgery, immobilization, loss of vision, and eventual loss of my left eye. During this so-called tragic event, my grandson and I were bonded together for our joint healing, even though we did not name it as such.

As mentioned in chapter 11, as part of our shared healing needs, he spent time with me, just being there, reading to me, doing art, talking, and "hanging out," so to speak. During this time, I was confined to lying on my stomach on a massage table 24 hours a day, with 15-minute breaks only, with my head down in the cradle.

As the summer months passed, from June into August, with this prolonged confinement and hoped-for-healing, it became increasingly evident that my eye could not be saved, in spite of my yielding to the quiet, the prone position, the healing rituals, and so on. The retina of the eye seemed to be reattaching, but the pressure was not returning to my eye. I had to remain with my head down, but as late August approached, I was now able to be up from my confinement for longer periods of time. While it had not been confirmed yet, I sensed that the inevitable was upon us and I would indeed lose my eye. At the same time, a new season of time and life was upon us as a family.

I anticipated my grandson returning to school and a new cycle of time emerging. I suggested we do a healing ritual together. I felt that we both needed to somehow ground and concretize the trauma and shock, pain, guilt, and loss we were both experiencing in our own ways. So, I mentioned us doing a healing ritual before his school started, so we could have a turning point in the experience. I asked him what he thought we should do. *"Should we bury something? Should we draw something? Should we burn something?"* What did he think?

So, after a week or so of thinking about it, one day he said: *"Gigi, I know what we can do for a ritual .... We can bury some of the quartz rock stones you have under your massage table; we can do it outside where the accident occurred. It is just a suggestion."* I said *"Oh, Demitri, I think that is an excellent suggestion and the perfect ritual for us to do."* (Under my head cradle on the massage table, I had a basket of rose quartz stones that was a collection from my husband. As he took his daily hikes in the mountain trails a couple of blocks from our home, he always picked up natural rose quartz stones and brought them back to me for my basket; these stones were something to look at as I lay face down. I also had a basket of rose petals under my head cradle, along with the basket of rose quartz; these petals were a collection from the many loving bouquets of roses that had been sent to me).

I exclaimed to Demitri that I thought his ideas were perfect, and I suggested we add the rose petals to the rose quartz stones, to offer a blessing to the ritual to put on top of the burial. So, we each picked three rose quartz stones to bury (I don't know how we decided on three; it seems instinctive) and took the basket of rose petals to the side lawn where the accident occurred. I identified the spot where I thought the accident occurred, but he very quickly said, *"No, it is here"* (a foot or so away from the spot I chose). So, I said *"Oh, OK."*

We then proceeded to dig our holes to bury our stones on the site of the accident. (In the meantime, a lone deer had entered the back part of the large lawn, standing among the trees, watching over us like a lone mystical guardian in the midst of our healing pain.) Just as we were preparing to bury our stones, I asked him if there was anything he wanted to say about the stones he was burying; what feelings he was burying with the stones.

In taking each stone, one by one, he said the following: *Well, with the first stone, I am burying that I am sorry I didn't tell you I was going to swing the club when I did; for the second stone, I am sorry that the club hit your eye; for the third stone, the same: I am sorry that I hit your eye."* Then he buried each of the three stones.

Then I took my three stones and told him that I really did not expect him to tell me he was going to swing, because there was no way he could know that I was coming toward him to help him with his swing. (This was the first time he had conveyed the guilt he must have felt about not letting me know he was going to swing, harboring some of the feelings that it was his fault). I explained to him it was not his fault, nor my fault, that it was one of those uncanny accidents and mysteries of life that just happened and we were learning about together.

Then I buried my stone, and explained what I was burying with my stones: *For my first stone, I am burying my forgiveness of myself for getting in your line of fire with the golf club and causing so much pain for all of us; for the second stone, I am burying forgiveness of you for the fact that it happened; and for the third stone, forgiveness of the situation.*

Then, after we had covered up the stones with dirt and grass, I suggested that we bless our ritual and our requests by sprinkling rose petals over the site. So, we each took a handful of rose petals and scattered them over our burial sites for our stones, which were side by side, but not touching. Then, very spontaneously, just as we were almost through, Demitri said: *"Wait!"* Then he took the rest of the rose petals from the basket and spread them all over the two sites, making it one spot. Then he said: *"Now we are joined."* This story of practicing forgiveness, which accompanied a shared healing ritual, was a special, significant event and dramatic turning point for this moment in our time and experience. Giving voice and concrete action to the forgiveness that was lying dormant in our healing process became necessary to allow the situation to turn from a tragedy into a shared blessing and connection around life's journey we share.

REMEMBERING CONTINUING

During my own personal healing journey, and during my felt tragedy, one of the felt-miracles for me was a sense of wonder and gratitude for all the love and blessings that surrounded me. I was almost overcome with the sense of having everything I needed for my experience; for example, not only the love, support, and healing energy/actions of my family, close friends, colleagues, neighbors, and so on, but a sense of awe and gratitude for my home, the layout of the rooms; the fact that everything was just as it needed to be to contribute to my healing. Walking to a separate bathroom that was down the hall from my bedroom, instead of using the master bathroom, not only gave my husband and me some needed space for the different treatments and uses of the bathrooms, but making a spare bathroom my own, during this time, gave me just the right amount of exercise I needed for my 15-minute breaks from the massage table. In the short walk down the upstairs hallway, I again became highly conscious of and grateful for the fact that I could see and appreciate the view of the house, the outdoor, the flow of the space, the rich opulence of the carpets we had purchased together years ago in Morocco, the rich grain of the hardwood floors, the light on the staircase, the fact that I could WALK, that I could SEE, all became great sources of awe, wonder, gratitude, and humility for me. So, in becoming grounded to the present now, in surrendering to the moment, seeing it through eyes of love, wonder, forgiveness, gratitude, and surrender changed my tragedy into a sacred gift, a blessing of appreciation and humility at the same time. I began to deeply appreciate and honor the fact that I felt I was being held in grace, mercy, and abiding love throughout the entire process of my accident, treatment, recovering, and healing.

I continue to this day to be in awe at all the blessings that surround me, even when I am most despairing or alone. I continually give thanks. As wise sages remind us: Bless and forgive everything. May every breath be a prayer.

These are my mantras to this day. And at this very moment, I reside in a deep place of gratitude and surrender with where I am here in México, writing this book, being able to see; to type; to have a computer; to see the blue sea, the sparkling sun reflecting on the water; to hear the sounds of osprey cheeping and circling around me outside my door. I sometimes become overwhelmed by gratitude and deep surrender. I am reminded of the Biblical quote: *"Do you not know it is God's good pleasure to give you the Kingdom of God, and all its glory"* and then I remember, and give thanks again. I continually bow down.

Another personal experience of remembering with *Gratitude* and with *Surrendering* was the very accident itself and the fact that I had to hold my head down to allow reattachment of the retina. At first, I was so weak it didn't matter to me, as I was fully and completely surrendering to what was upon me to do. During my surgeries, I felt total peace because I indeed had to surrender to others and their skills and treatments.

But as I was able to be up more from "my cradle," I still had to hold my head down; I felt humiliated and embarrassed, as if I had to hold my head in shame of some kind. I kept thinking of the Kingston Trio song: "Hang down your head Tom Dooley," as if I had done something terribly wrong. But after a short while of holding my head down, I realized that I was not holding my head down in shame and humiliation, but rather, in holding my head down, I was looking down; I was looking inward with gratitude, with reverence, still with humility, but with a different sense of awe and thankfulness. I began to think of myself as *"Bowing Down"* in silence, with deep gratitude and surrender, for all that I had and for all that I was experiencing, for all I was given as a great gift/blessing from this so-called tragedy.

This ongoing practice of gratitude and surrendering was/is part of my ongoing healing, my re-patterning, helping me toward my evolving experiencing/returning to/remembering the Infinity of Universal Love.

Hence, one of the reasons for writing this book is not only to write what I am continuing to learn, and need to learn, but also to hope that someone else may understand and be touched; someone else may share these insights and embark on our common path toward Love. Realizing that ultimately it is through forgiveness, giving gratitude, and bowing down with surrender to life itself, that it is a movement toward the highest level of consciousness—a level of consciousness I/we all seek at some deep level.

Deepening the Meanings of the Sacred Circle of Life-Death: Personal Remembering

To continue to share part of my own learning/healing journey as part of the experiential discovery of a living Caring Science, I turn to my most extreme personal pain and suffering as my lessons for grasping deeper meaning of the life-death cycle for myself and others; realizing the mystery that holds its own pattern and rhythm for each of us. This insight and deeper meaning came not from our established religious teachings, although it can be found there intellectually. My personal learning of deeper meaning of life-death also did not come from philosophical texts or from reading sacred ancient texts, but lessons can certainly be learned that way.

Rather, it was and continues to be the personal, experiential living, *Being, Becoming*—going through a tragic, sudden life crisis that brought my deepest knowing. This experiential reality of facing my pain and shock of loss came with the unexpected and sudden death of my husband through suicide; this came after he took loving care of me during my eye injury and healing. Such a horror can only be lived through; one learns how to bear the unbearable when faced with such shock and deep loss. However, my living and facing the horrible and holy nature of it was softened and expanded by the teachings of a Native American Elder, Black Wolf.

Some know my personal story or at least part of it. I have found that the more I heal, the more able I am to share my story. I have shared part of this with groups over the past 3 years or so. My story is one of learning very deeply from a new lens, literally and figuratively, through new eyes, the great mystery of life-death. Wisdom was conveyed to me from a wise elder, a Spirit guide of sorts, a Native American Elder, Black Wolf, who consoled me and gave me a picture of the infinity and vastness of meaning, way beyond my limited earth plane view. He may not even know how significant his teaching was for me.

Black Wolf brought deeper meaning to my suffering and pain by telling the story of his people's cosmology. He put it somewhat this way as I recall our conversation: (Black Wolf, 1999, personal communication, Cambridge, England).

> We all come from the Spirit world. We come here to this Earth Plane for a specific purpose to complete our soul's journey. We choose when we come and for what purpose. Our purpose may be very grand; it may be very small. It may be as simple as being at a certain place at a certain time to assist someone in crossing the street. But, when our soul's purpose has been

completed and we are spiritually satisfied we return home to the Spirit world. In other words, when Father Spirit calls, we return home to the Spirit world from which we came. The Spirit world is Universal Love. One of the reasons we all love new babies is because they are fresh from the Spirit world and Universal Love. It is also a reason to honor our elders because they are preparing to return to the Spirit world.

I then asked Black Wolf, "What if someone returns home prematurely?" (wanting to be discreet about my husband's death.) He said; *"What do you mean prematurely? That is your word?"*

I said, "Well, like suicide for example." Then he said, *"Well, in our cosmology, we do not have a word for suicide"* and repeated: *"When someone's soul purpose is done, and they are spiritually satisfied, they return home to the spirit world. When Grandfather spirit calls we have to go."*

What becomes/became so meaningful for me is that after he said this, I flashed back on a moment when my husband was taking intense care of me and giving me a full body massage. Out of the blue, it seems, he said to me, while giving me this loving massage: "I feel like I have been preparing all my life, just for this; just to be here to take care of you."

I remember at the time when he said this, I thought it was the most beautiful, loving expression; I was touched with his tenderness and spontaneity to say something so sweetly. However, in retrospect, another whole meaning and deep sense of peace crashed into my head and heart, and I grasped my husband's death/suicide from a very different perspective.

Black Wolf's vision and cosmology of life-death, combined with the actual experience I had with my husband, literally transformed me on the spot and gave me a deep sense of peace and meaning. His call to return home to the Spirit world, his task being completed, all took on entirely new and different meanings for me. It had cosmic meaning beyond anything that I/we can understand from our limited view of physical life alone.

On this life journey, we all come face to face with mysteries and unknowns, and all are challenged to find our way. My story may not have meaning for anyone else, but it is a story about how each of us has to find our own meaning about life and death that is congruent for our self and our situation. However, it seems that usually any truly lasting deeper meaning-making invites and enters into the sacred, silent Infinity, that ineffable place of unknowns, while simultaneously offering us a greater sense of purpose in the infinite scheme of the great sacred circle of life-death. This, too, is our ongoing task to deepen and evolve our humanity toward our higher/the highest consciousness, which is love; with Love comes forgiveness and freedom from self-imposed suffering. The result is a continuing search to inner life and its intersection with the Infinite, as part of the earth plane spiritual journey: to grow in Love, compassion, and caring. Through this experience, I learned once more to surrender, to *Become Love* again.

Understand that anyone's story could be my story, and my story could be anyone else's story. You and I share this journey of evolving our humanity toward more and more Love and Light. But, first, we become Love and Light for our self. How else can we engage in Caring-Healing practices in our work, our world, and our science?

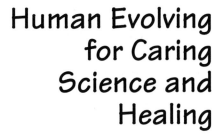

19

Human Evolving
for Caring
Science and
Healing

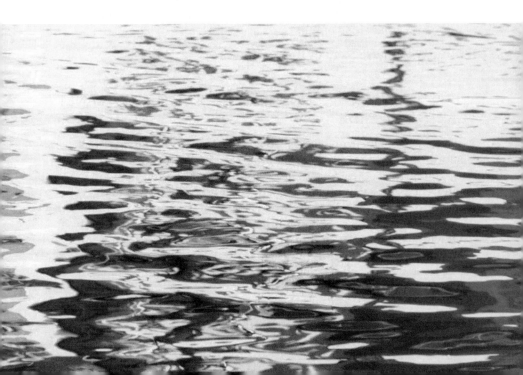

It seems to me that one of the reasons we have been limited and restricted in our human evolution, in the ways we have defined ourselves, our jobs, and our science is because we have failed to see that work in the field of caring-healing intersects with the very tasks of not only "facing our humanity," but deepening our humanity. Indeed, the very endeavors we are embarked upon with respect to being human are the very endeavors we mirror, reflect, and engage in as part of our caring-healing work with self and other. Just what are these human tasks that intersect with the Caring Science model? Well, the three tasks just discussed above include some of our essential human tasks toward healing: *Forgiveness, Offering Gratitude, and Surrendering.*

There are at least four or five other more abstract human endeavors we all share in our humanity as well as our common work, regardless of professional/personal background. We may not even be aware that these are the activities we are engaged in until they are brought to our conscious attention and awareness. These endeavors include at least the following challenges for locating our work, our science, and our human evolution within Caring Science: (Watson, *Journal of Advanced Nursing*, 2002).

- ❋ Healing our relationship with Self /Other/Planet Earth/Universe;

- ❋ Understanding and transforming our own and other's suffering;

- ❋ Deepening and expanding our understanding of living and dying; acknowledging the shadow-light cycle of the great sacred circle of life;

- ❋ Preparing for our own death.

HEALING OUR RELATIONSHIP WITH SELF/OTHER/PLANET EARTH/UNIVERSE

Within this framework, we now realize more than ever that before we can engage in healing practices, including medical and nursing practice, we have to deal with healing our relationship with self and Other, in that it all begins with self and radiates out to the universe. Within the field of health care, and nursing in particular, there is a long history of being unkind, if not cruel, among ourselves; likewise, there are stories and research studies that condemn medical education and authoritarian practices that perpetuate unkind, cruel and, in some instances, abusive practices in health professional education and practice field. Yet, we are charged with moral and social expectations to *care* and to be *healers*.

This focus on healing our relationships becomes very personal, yet it impacts, if not informs, our professional practices. This basic task of being human and becoming more humane intersects with our professional focus in caring-healing. We forget that our health care work is greater than we have acknowledged; the human nature of our work has been too small and limited in its scope in relation to the rich, complex nature of this deeply human work.

To engage in healing our self and our relationship with each other and beyond, the practices of *Forgiveness, Offering Gratitude, and Surrendering* to higher/deeper sources for consolation, creativity, insight, and heart-centered action is a way to begin. It seems that our relationship with our self is most critical to all other aspects of healing work, including our own personal health. It starts with self and moves in concentric radiating circles out to all whom we touch physically, locally, non-locally, and energetically. We return again and again to these basic human practices to stay alive, awake, and to sustain our humanity. As Rumi put it:

> . . . It doesn't matter that you've broken
> your vow a thousand times, still
> come, and yet again, come.
> (2001, p. 225)

AND his reminder/rejoinder for our living/Being/Becoming:

> . . . Don't pretend to know
> something you haven't experienced.
> There's a necessary dying.
> . . . Be ground. Be crumbled, so wildflowers will come up
> where you are. You've been
> stony for too many years. Try something different. Surrender.
> Rumi, 2001

BETTERING OUR UNDERSTANDING OF HUMAN SUFFERING: HELPING TO TRANSFORM ITS MEANING IN (OUR) LIFE

It is widely held that to be human is to suffer. All major religions and wisdom traditions and text deal with suffering in one way or another. One of our human tasks at the individual and collective level is to make meaning of our own suffering; to take it from the abstract concept into our daily lives when we are actually witnessing and experiencing our own and others' real, overt suffering. Indeed, if we had no suffering, there would be no depth to us as humans, no humility, no compassion (Tolle, 2003). It is our suffering that cracks the ego shell and therefore has a necessary purpose in helping us surrender to what is, and is necessary until we realize it is unnecessary (Tolle, 2003).

However, we also know from our human experiences that we can find new meanings and that we seek meaning to assist us when we are most vulnerable, fearful, and "suffering" the slings and arrows known as life. It seems we learn through the deeply personal encounters with suffering that we learn we cannot go around life, we have to go through the experience in order to not only survive, but to thrive, to sustain a sense of hope for continued existence, living. Perennial philosophies and sacred teachings inform us repeatedly that true freedom and the end of suffering is living in such a way that we surrender to what is, and in such a way as if you had completely chosen whatever you feel or experience at this moment; that is, "this inner alignment with NOW is the end of suffering" (Tolle, 2003, p. 118).

However, suffering is both necessary and unnecessary. We are informed both by our experiences of suffering and our testing of how to live as well as by our sacred texts for how to live. For example, as long as we adhere to a fixed, solid, physical dimension as all there is to life, then we are locked into concrete psyche and physical pain, generating an interpretation or story that makes us unhappy. It seems that suffering begins when we mentally name or label a situation in some way as undesirable or bad, which then personalizes it and brings a reactive ego response to the situation. Naming something as bad causes an emotional contraction within us. When we surrender, let it be, without congealing it, fixing it, naming it as negative, then enormous power is suddenly available to us, beyond suffering (Tolle, 2003, p. 122).

Tolle (1999, 2003), in his contemporary writings, as well as ancient Buddhist texts remind us that all suffering is ego-centered and due to resistance. For example, the Buddha's basic philosophy was considered with inner transformation by achieving insight into the "Four Noble Truths" of Buddhism: (Solomon & Higgins, 1997, p. 19):

1. Life is suffering;

2. Suffering arises from selfish craving;

3. Selfish craving can be eliminated;

4. One can eliminate selfish craving by following the right way.

The right way to liberation, enlightenment, or elimination/transformation of suffering is called the *Eightfold path* of Buddhism, which consists of (1) right seeing, (2) right thinking; (3) right speech; (4) right action; (5) right effort, (6) right living; (7) right mindfulness; and (8) right meditation (Solomon & Higgins, 1997, p. 19).

These are big orders for how to live a life that is full of suffering due to impermanence, when we cling for permanence and delude ourselves that there is a permanent self and permanency of life. At another level, suffering is a result of our craving for separateness, for our individuality, our independence, separating and distancing ourselves from each other, other human beings, as well as from our environment, our world, our universe. This, too, contributes to human suffering according to contemporary science as well as ancient sacred texts.

This underlying reality of impermanence is tied up with our avoidance of participating in the cyclical nature of all of life and of the law of impermanence of all things. That is, underneath what is perceived as fixed and unchanging reveals itself as a living paradox, a yin-yang, *both-and* phenomena. Underneath the felt suffering and pain, there resides an abiding presence, the infinity of universal Love as a field that offers an abiding peace, an unchanging deep stillness, an uncaused joy that transcends good and bad, pain and no-pain (Tolle, 1999). This underneath abiding field that holds us in the midst of the constant movement is what T.S. Eliot named *"the still point."*

At the big-picture level, this impermanence cycle mirrors the great circle of birth-death; creation-destruction, growth-dissolution, manifest-un-manifest fields. In this way of understanding change and impermanence, everything is rising up and falling away; expanding and contracting, mirroring the breath and rhythm of life's natural energetic processes in all things.

Buddha made this discovery the very heart of his teaching: the cyclical nature and impermanence of the universe. Everything is in constant flux. Our challenge to find new understanding about the nature of human suffering is not only all of our human tasks, it is a professional task in that for a caring-healing practitioner/scientist the two intersect. And as we seek new understandings that deepen our humanity, we become more humane, compassionate, wise, and healing in our work and world. Our task as health and caring-healing profes-sionals is to realize that in both our science world and our practice world, our work and jobs have been too narrow for the deep human nature of the work that we really are confronted with in our caring-healing relationships with self, others, and our universe. A reality to live is to find the still point, in the midst of the law of constant change; to find the abiding peace and presence of divine intelligence, a universal field of Love that transcends all the felt change that we solidify and freeze in our experience, contributing to more pain, more suffering. But in the deeper wisdom/understanding and experiencing that can take us *beyond-suffering,* we suddenly realize that there is a marked difference between pain with suffering and pain without suffering. It is how we perceive and allow the impermanence to move through us, not clinging, freezing, and fixing the temporary condition or circumstance in our mind, our bodies, emotions, or even our hearts.

In the end, we are always "in training" and if and when we practice this understanding and acceptance of suffering, we learn to transform that suffering into hope, love, and deep compassion. (Thich Nhat Hanh, 2003). As Thich Nhat Hanh (2003) reminds us, the foundation of hope, love, and compassion is already there in our hearts and minds, awaiting our entering this new place of consciousness and learning to dwell there, thus transforming suffering into a deeper level of living.

Suffering

One way is to grasp the reality of suffering and learn at a personal level how new insights can change our views, if not transform our views of life. This change happened to me at a personal experiential level when I had my eye injury and was experiencing acute and what was unbearable pain at the time. I learned the difference between having pain with suffering and having pain without suffering. I learned this through the practice of deep meditation whereby I was able to witness my pain and watch it as a continuous movement-of-energy, rising up and falling away; it was when I resisted the pain and solidified or fixed it that it congealed, so to speak, and became more painful and brought more suffering, both physically and emotionally. So, at a physical level of experience, I learned to meditate my way through a great deal of the pain, or at least catch myself when I was resisting. In opening my self to the experience itself, as a witness of my own experience, the pain passed through me energetically, in waves of energy, expanding and contracting. It was the contracting and congealing that brought the most suffering, but by watching it move beyond, and through, me; by staying still with the process, it became some sort of a miracle. That is only one small example of physical pain, but the same process can be explored and discovered for other forms of pain, psychic, emotional, mental, which also came as part of my own journey toward healing.

DEEPENING AND EXPANDING OUR UNDERSTANDING OF LIVING AND DYING; ACKNOWLEDGING THE SHADOW/LIGHT CYCLE OF THE GREAT SACRED CIRCLE OF LIFE

While we adhere to health and curing/caring and healing as our primary mission in this health care work, we also now have to acknowledge honestly that we work within the great circle of life-death. This reality recognizes that we all share this common task of facing our humanity at a deep level, both personally and professionally. What we do is not without consequences, in that one way or another we are contributing to and co-participating with the web of life. In all of our work and actions we are working within the universal energy field of infinity that enfolds and surrounds and upholds all of life—time, past, present, future; time before and time after the earth plane of existence; spirit transcending physical body transcending death as we know it. So, making and seeking meaning about understanding and deepening our view and appreciation for all of life is part of our human quest. David Bohm proposed that *meaning is a form of Being* (Weber, 1986, p. 18); that is, it is realizing that through our meanings we change nature's being. Human's meaning-making capacity turns us into nature's partner, in shaping our evolution. Bohm suggests that what we are actually doing by engaging in dialogue with the cosmos is changing its idea of itself (Weber, 1986). This perspective is quite awesome and humbling to consider the majesty of the universe and our relationship with it in a deeper way.

Renee Weber believes this deeper dimension is activated in all the participants through dialogue; it is through engagement and dialogue whereby our own world-line/song-line intersects with and forms part of the process. This song-line of relationship and intersecting web of life continues and carries over from the cosmos into our own spiritual journey (Weber, 1986, p. 18).

Part of this meaning making for a great depth of life-death and our place within it is related to an awakening: awakening to the fact that we are Spirit made whole in physical manifestation. As Teilhard de Chardin noted: we are not just physical beings having a spiritual experience; rather we are spiritual beings having a physical experience. This perspective now converges with language such as manifest and non-manifest field of existence. This view of awakening seeks to honor the unknown, the unseen as much as the seen; often realizing the illusion of what we think we know and see on the physical plane to *be* true reality. Just as in exploring deeper dimensions of suffering, we learn that what we perceive as suffering, at one level, is our own congealing and freezing of the divine flow of life energy; in other words, not being in flow with natural laws of nature and natural timeless rhythm of all things in the universe: the seasons, the tides, the cycles of time and existence; the coming into being of living creatures and the passing out of being on physical plane existence, be it human or other living things. Everything is constantly changing and deepening our understanding of this mystery of life, coming and going in our midst, including our own.

Preparing for Our Own Death

When you see and accept the impermanent nature of all life forms,
a strange sense of peace comes upon you.
Tolle, 2003, p. 105

Another final human task we all share, which intersects with the nature of caring-healing work, is coming face-to-face in preparing for our own death. As the sages say, without honoring death, we are not fully alive. Indeed, in the cosmic sense again, we are dying every moment, in that with each breath we experience the miracle of life itself and the precious, yet delicate, nature of how we are held in the hands of that which is greater than us. And at a deeper metaphysical or metaphorical level or within Native American cosmology or any indigenous belief system, death is not the end, it is a continuation of the sacred wheel of life. And as the expression goes: Who is to say that life is not death, and death is not life? And we certainly glimpse situations in which we are called to ask about the living dead we sometimes feel in our hearts and/or in our midst. In preparing for our death, we learn from those who are our teachers along the way. Those who are undergoing the life-death transition can be a gift for our learning and preparation. They can teach us if we listen and are able to be present to their experience and be there with and for them as we are able.

When working with others during times of despair, vulnerability, and unknowns, we are challenged to learn again, to re-examine our own meaning of life and death. As we do so, we engage in more authentic process and practices to cultivate and sustain caring-healing for self and others. Such care and practices elicit and call upon profound wisdom and understanding, beyond knowledge, that touch and draw upon the human heart and soul. However, this learning can be informed by our science, a science that honors the whole. A Science of Caring that opens to the infinity of our learning and evolving. Death is not an anomaly or the most horrible of all events as our culture has us believe, but as Tolle reminds us, the most natural thing in the world (Tolle, 2003). "Is there anything that is not subject to birth and death, anything that is eternal?" (Tolle, 2003, p. 109).

In this reminder of heart-centered knowing and wisdom beyond words and conventional knowledge, our basic humanness transcends circumstances, time, and place. Our being and becoming more humane and evolved allows us to engage once again in compassionate service and science, motivated by love, both human and Cosmic. From this place of deepening our humanity, we offer to our self, and those whom we meet on our path, our compassionate response for fulfilling our chosen life's work and calling. In encountering and facing death of self and others, we are in sacred space, touching the mystery of life itself, dwelling in the space of Infinity.

Just as it is in our personal lives during crises or illness, tragedy, loss, or impending death, we ponder spiritual questions that go beyond the physical material world; it is here in our evolving professional-scientific life that we may need to ponder new meaning. In our conventional, dispirited, physical-technical life form, deathbed of sorts, Caring Science offers new freedom, new space to reconsider a deeper meaning of caring-healing work and phenomena.

It is here in our wounded, broken science models that a Caring Science can reorient us or, at least, point us toward another science model that may be more hopeful for understanding and living our caring and healing. It is here, in this transition, this space and place between the breaths, that we can quiet the pace, bow down, and take in new energy and new directions to inspire our work and our world. The more science learns, it seems the greater nature and life's mystery grows. As we seek to increase our knowledge and wisdom of our deepening and expanding humanity, it opens science to even more profound beauty and wonder of life's infinite cosmic connectedness and oneness in which we reside (Weber, 1986).

So, within Caring Science, we now have a new call to bring us back to that which already resides deep within us and intersects with the focus of caring and healing at this time. It allows us to uncover the latent infinite Love in our work and world and connect with contemporary philosophies that invite Love and Caring through our ethics of Being and Becoming and Belonging. This text invites us to make the leap of faith back into metaphysics and a moral foundation for our science and our life, to incorporate into our science the reverence for the sacredness of life and death and our shared human heart-centered evolution.

Ultimately and finally, may we be inspired with a renewed commitment *to remember* who we are and why we came here: *To Love, To Serve, and To Remember.*

Afterword: Caring and Peace

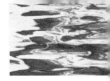

I find it ironical that, over these past few years, I have been given the gift of Spirit—the opportunity to fully experience life and spirit in raw form, in the midst of deep suffering, pain, isolation, abandonment, and despair, but also joy, peace, and love beyond measure. The lesson, as Buddha reminded us: It does not matter how long we have forgotten, only how soon we *remember*.

It is as if we sometimes have to be stopped in order to allow our souls/our soulful purpose in our personal/professional life to catch up with us. This moment may be one of transition/transformation for us as individuals as well as for the professions. It may be fresh; it may be dull. It may be a crossroads for our survival if we are to *remember* our humanity and its deep connection with caring-healing work.

When we evolve toward higher consciousness that embraces Caring in the deepest sense of Caritas/Love, both human and Cosmic, that comes from heart-centered living and practicing, we are contributing holographically to the evolution of humanity, helping to sustain caring in instances where it is threatened. We do this through our heart-centered consciousness, integrating head and heart into our very presence as we radiate our Love into the infinity of the universe, affecting the whole: the collective consciousness of the world. So, one person's healing, one person's caring is contributing to the caring and healing of the world.

Caring/Love radiates in concentric circles from self, to Other, to Community, to Planet Earth, to Infinity of the Universe. As there is an increase in Love/Caring in the world, there is a higher evolution of human consciousness affecting the whole. Caring/Love begets more caring/love, whereas a lack of Caring/Love begets a lack of caring/love. There is a relationship between Caring and Peace, in that a lack of Caring/Love manifests in non-caring behaviors, violence, dehumanization, alienation, a "totalizing"/objectifying of other as non-human, therefore, allowing us to do things to other as objects, not as fully humans.

As we move forward into this new millennium, we face the challenges of how to bring contemplative values and practices into our everyday life as well as our science. As posed by Jon Kabat-Zinn, it is now time for society to turn attention toward what is referred to "inner technologies," to become more contemplative, mindful, caring, and compassionate. To move forward in this new era, we have to become more conscious, more intentional about this perspective.

This inner technology has meditation, another Caring Science strategy, as its center and is the one form that has the capacity to elevate our consciousness (Kabat-Zinn, 1997, p. 259) for more caring, harmony, and Love among humanity, transcending nationalities, borders, and boundaries that keep humanity separate from each other.

As we evolve and attend to more fully developing and expanding a model of Caring Science, we are also contributing to evolution of a moral community that is based on common human bonds of trust and love, not fear. So, there is an increasing need to acknowledge the relationship between caring/love and peace in our lives and our world. This work toward cultivation of inner technologies becomes a form of ontological evolution for our humanity.

It starts within the individual heart of each of us. This work is an invitation, an evocation, a call to enter into this space where there are new possibilities for shaping our lives, our work, and our world as we move forward into this new world. May we tread consciously and intentionally with love and light in our hearts and actions? May we, once again, be reminded *"we help to shape another's world, not by theories and views but by our very being and attitude toward him. Herein lies the unarticulated and one might say anonymous demand that we take care of life which trust has placed in our hands"* (Logstrup, 1997, p. 19).

I close with the Chinese proverb I frequently recite because it captures the relationship between our light, caring, and peace in the world:

> If there is light in the soul,
> There is beauty in the person.
> If there is beauty in the person,
> There is harmony in the house.
> If there is harmony is the house,
> There is order in the nation.
> If there is order in the nation,
> There will be peace in the world.
> (Ancient Chinese Proverb: Anonymous)

Closing Meditation:
Mantra for Self and Others

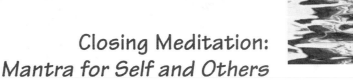

The breeze at dawn has secrets to tell you
Don't go back to sleep.
You must ask for what you really want
Don't go back to sleep.
People are going back and forth across the doorsill
Where the two worlds touch.
The door is round and open.
Don't go back to sleep.

Rumi, 2001

Table CM-1

Table of Major Philosophies Underpinning Caring Science

PHILOSOPHER:	PRIMARY FOCUS	PRIMARY SOURCE CITATION
Emmanuel Levinas Born 1906 in Lithuania; from 1923 on lived in France rest of his life; held several university posts in philosophy in France; Died in Paris, 1995	"Ethics of face"; Belonging to Infinity of Universal Love Before Ontology of Being; Ethics and Philosophy as "first principle" and starting point for science; Humanity is sustained by facing our own and other's humanity; vs. totalizing our humanness.	Levinas, E. *Totality and Infinity*. Duquesne University. Pittsburgh, PA, 1969. 14th printing. 2000. Critchley, S. & Bernasconi, R. (Eds) (2002). *The Cambridge Companion to Levinas*. Cambridge: Cambridge Press.
Knud Logstrup Born 1905 in Copenhagen; studied in Copenhagen and France; Professor of Ethics and Philosophy: Univ. of Aarhus, Denmark; died 1981	"The ethical demand" we "hold another person in our *Hands*"; Logstrup removes human as sovereign controller of the university; The basic expression of life is to both give and receive. The True sovereign expressions of life are expressive actions and attitudes of trust, honesty, fidelity, love, caring. forgiveness, etc.	Logstrup, K. E. (1997). *The Ethical Demand*. Notre Dame: Notre Dame University, 1997. Logstrup, K. E. (1995). *Metaphysics. Vol. I.* Milwaukee, Marquette Univ.

Appendices Introduction

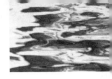

Selected Essays/Contributing Chapters Reflective of Caring Science Model

1. Quinn, J., Smith, M., Ritenbaugh, C., Swanson, K., & Watson, J. (2003). Research guidelines for assessing the impact of the healing relationship in clinical nursing. Reprinted with permission from *Alternative Therapies in Health and Medicine,* 9(3)(Suppl), A65–A79.
2. Watson, J. (2002). Intentionality and caring-healing consciousness: A practice of transpersonal nursing. Reprinted with permission from *Journal of Holistic Nursing Practice,* 16(4), 12–19.
3. Watson, J. (2000). Leading via caring-healing: The fourfold way toward transformative leadership. Reprinted with permission from *Nursing Administrative Quarterly,* 25(1), 1–6.
4. Watson, J. (2003). Love and caring: Ethics of face and hand. Reprinted with permission from *Nursing Administrative Quarterly,* 27(3), 197–202.
5. Watson, J. (2002). Metaphysics of virtual caring communities. Reprinted with permission from *International Journal of Human Caring,* 6(1), 41–45.
6. Watson, J., & Smith, M. (2002). Caring science and the science of unitary human beings: A trans-theoretical discourse. Reprinted with permission from *Journal of Advanced Nursing,* 37(5), 452-461.

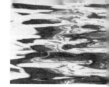

Research Guidelines for Assessing the Impact of the Healing Relationship in Clinical Nursing*

Janet F. Quinn, PhD, RN, FAAN; Marlaine Smith, PhD, RN;
Cheryl Ritenbaugh, PhD, MPH; Kristen Swanson, PhD, RN, FAAN;
and Jean Watson, PhD, RN, HNC, FAAN

Janet F. Quinn is Associate Professor, adjoint; Marlaine Smith is Associate Professor and Associate Dean of Academic Programs; and M. Jean Watson is Distinguished Professor, Endowed Chair in Caring Science, University of Colorado Health Sciences Center, School of Nursing, Denver. Cheryl Ritenbaugh is Senior Investigator, Kaiser Permanente Center for Health Research, Portland, Oregon. Kristen Swanson is Professor and Chair, Family and Child Nursing, University of Washington School of Nursing, Seattle.

The term *healing relationship* has been defined by the Samueli Institute for Information Biology (SUB) consensus group as "the quality and characteristics of interactions between healer and healee that facilitate healing. Characteristics of this interaction involve empathy, caring, love, warmth, trust, confidence, credibility, honesty, expectation, courtesy, respect, and communication."[1] Combining elements of this definition with the SUB definition of healing gives a fuller sense of the concept: "Those physical, mental, social, and spiritual processes of recovery, repair, renewal, and transformation that increase wholeness. . . . Healing is an emergent process of the whole system, and may or may not involve curing."[1]

If the relationship between practitioner and client, between healer and healee, is in fact a variable in healing, then whatever is healing in that relationship warrants rigorous discernment. Furthermore, because the role of healer is not specific to gender or discipline, guidelines for inquiry into healing relationships must transcend disciplinary boundaries. Nevertheless, each discipline brings its own focus

*Quinn, J., Smith, M., Ritenbaugh, C., Swanson, K., & Watson, J. (2003). Research guidelines for assessing the impact of the healing relationship in clinical nursing. Reprinted with permission from *Alternative Therapies in Health and Medicine,* 9(3)(Suppl), A65–A79.

and way of conceptualizing this relationship and thus contributes a unique perspective. The American Nurses Association has long defined nursing as the assessment, diagnosis, and treatment of human responses to actual and potential health problems, combining the art of caring and the science of health care.[2] Nursing is grounded in the philosophy and science of human caring,[3] with its purpose being to "put the patient in the best condition for nature to act upon him."[4]

The purpose of this Appendix is to explore the healing relationship through the disciplinary lens of nursing and to propose guidelines for research methodologies that might help to elucidate both the process and outcomes of healing relationships in clinical nursing practice. These guidelines might be applied to research on the impact of healing relationships between clients and other health professionals as well. The checklist at the end of this Appendix summarizes the quality guidelines.

Rationale for Studying the Healing Relationship in Clinical Nursing Practice

Across disciplines, there exists both theoretical and empirical support for the claim that the relationship between clinicians and their patients is an important component of practice. What is not uniform across disciplines is the relative emphasis on this relationship as being integral to both the processes and outcomes of practice. In nursing, a focus on the whole person and the relationship between nurse and patient are central and primary. There are at least six cogent reasons for studying the healing relationship in nursing:

1. If the healing relationship is a factor in the outcomes of both conventional and complementary therapies, then nurses, as the largest group of health care professionals, are in key positions to add that element where it is missing and sustain it where it exists.

2. Nursing as a profession is being challenged by a profound shortage that has dramatic implications for the health of the health care system.[5] One reason for the shortage is that nursing work forces have been downsized in uninformed attempts to save money. Perhaps it was unfortunate ignorance of the role of the nurse-patient relationship in healing that helped to create this problem. Research in this area might serve to ameliorate this situation.

3. Theoretical literature in nursing asserts an association between caring/healing relationships and healing outcomes. It is important to study these assertions through well-designed scientific inquiry employing multiple methodologies.

4. Outcomes-focused studies can provide a much-needed rationale for improving care practices.

5. The measurement of healing relationships is essential in documenting their occurrence, providing empirical evidence of their outcomes, and ultimately enabling the development of patient-oriented and family-oriented "report cards" about the quality of relationship-centered care as delivered by units or institutions.

6. Heuristically, outcomes studies can lead to the support, extension, or rejection of existing theories of the healing relationship and can stimulate further inquiry.

Questions for Research

The first step in conducting research on any topic is the identification of salient research questions. The broad overview question in consideration here is: What is the impact of the healing relationship in clinical nursing practice? Embedded in this question are dozens of other questions, many of which will require attention before the larger question can be answered. The following 20 are some of those questions, which do not exhaust the possible inquiries.

1. How can we assess "processes of recovery, repair, renewal and transformation that increase wholeness"?

2. If "healing is an emergent process of the whole system, and may or may not involve curing,"[1] how do we begin to assess the impact of the healing relationship on the whole system, including the clinician who is a part of that system?

3. What are the indicators of healing, particularly healing that does not include curing, and what are the appropriate measurements of these indicators?

4. How can we assess wholeness? How do we know it when we see it?

5. What are the essential mechanisms through which healing relationships are enacted?

6. What constitutes a "healing relationship" in the experience of both nurses and patients?

7. What are the necessary and sufficient elements that must be present in an interaction between people to make it a healing relationship?

8. How do participants in a healing relationship characterize both the process and its outcomes?

9. Do both members of the dyad concur on the essential elements or mechanisms through which healing is experienced?

10. Are there measurable indices of the occurrence of healing relationships?

11. Is time a necessary factor in the development and existence of a healing relationship, or can a healing relationship be constituted in one "caring moment"?

12. Is face-to-face proximity required for a healing relationship?

13. Can healing intentionality and energy be separated from the healing relationship?

14. Must both members of a dyad perceive the relationship as healing for it to be labeled as such, and is this related to outcome?

15. Can there be a healing relationship with a patient with whom there is no verbal communication, i.e., a comatose patient or a person with advanced Alzheimer's disease?

16. Is it still a healing relationship if there is no observable outcome other than the participants' claim that it was a healing relationship?

17. Which standard health-related outcomes are most influenced by the healing relationship?

18. If there is an impact on healing related to the healing relationship, what is its mechanism of action?

19. Can the capacity to form a healing relationship be taught, or is it a personality trait that is either present or absent?

20. With these questions in mind, what are the best methodologies for the study of healing relationships and their outcomes?

Review of the Literature

The term *healing relationship* is not a commonplace in the health profession literature, as a review in MEDLINE, CINAHL and PsychINFO demonstrates. Furthermore, of the 84 citations returned using this search term, only 12 were actually related to the relationship between clinician and patient, and of those 12, one was a dissertation using a heuristic, qualitative methodology[6]; none of the rest were data-based.[7–17] If, in fact, we look only for previous work on this topic that incorporates all of the concepts included in our definitions, it would be safe to say that the healing relationship is virtually unstudied, with the exception of a good deal of qualitative work in nursing, which will be reviewed below.

Review of the psychology literature using related terms such as *therapeutic relationship, therapeutic alliance, therapeutic bond, empathy,* and others, reveals thousands of articles and hundreds of outcomes studies over many years. This literature essentially concludes that the relationship between the therapist and the client is a stronger predictor of outcome than the actual type of therapy or the extent of the therapist's training.[18–22] A recent meta-analysis of 79 studies of the therapeutic alliance concluded that alliance is moderately related to outcomes of psychotherapy.[23] "The direct association between alliance and outcome identified in this empirical review is supportive of the hypothesis that the alliance may be therapeutic in and of itself. In other words, if a proper alliance is established between a patient and a therapist, the patient will experience the relationship as therapeutic, regardless of other psychological interventions."[23]

Almost exclusively limited to psychological symptoms and psychotherapeutic treatment approaches, this literature may provide some suggestive directions for our work but lacks a fundamental compatibility with our focus on the whole person in health and illness and with how clinical practice in nursing actually occurs. The difference between the therapist's weekly 1-hour session over many months and the nurse's intense but typically short-lived involvement is one clear example. Another is the access of the nurse to the body of the patient and the multitude of functions that touch fulfills in the nurse-patient relationship, from the most intimate of encounters in the bed bath to the simple act of holding a grieving parent.

In the medical and nursing literature, a search using the terms *healing relationship* and *outcomes* produced one article,[24] unrelated to our interest here. Searches using the terms *nurse-patient relationship, doctor-patient relationship, therapeutic relationship, patient-centered care, relationship-centered care,* and others, produced some outcomes studies.[25,26] The designs of these studies are typically interpretive, descriptive, or correlative, with few controlled trials. Dependent variables are almost exclusively limited to measures of patient satisfaction and compliance, but there is often a relationship between selected behaviors of health care clinicians and these outcomes. Kaplan, Greenfield, and Ware[27] reported data collected from four clinical trials that demonstrated that "better health," as measured physiologically (blood pressure and blood sugar), behaviorally (functional status), or more subjectively (evaluations of overall health status), was consistently related to specific aspects of physician-patient communication. In a few studies, some measure of symptom outcome[28] and functional status[29] is also included. Overall, the general suggestion of the literature is that various components of what one might consider to be healing relationships do appear to be related to at least some outcome measures. However, Mead and Bower, in summarizing the empirical literature on patient-centeredness, conclude that "the pattern of findings is somewhat inconsistent, particularly in relation to patient outcomes like health status or satisfaction" and that "it is likely that the more complex and contextual dimensions of patient-centeredness require development of new measures and analytic methods if further advances are to be made."[30]

The caring literature in nursing is closely aligned and consistent with the working definition of the healing relationship articulated by the Samueli Institute as well as with the SUB definition of healing. The art and science of human caring as developed within the discipline of nursing subsumes many related constructs, such as empathy, compassion, communication, instilling hope, trust, respect, love, patient-centeredness, and relationship-centeredness.

In 1999, Swanson synthesized the literature on caring in nursing science.[31] She reviewed 130 data-based articles, chapters, and books on caring published between 1980 and 1996. These included empirical and interpretive studies. The studies were categorized into the following five levels:

1. The capacity for caring (characteristics of caring persons)

2. Concerns and commitments (beliefs or values that underlie nurse caring)

3. Conditions (what affects, enhances, or inhibits the occurrence of caring)

4. Caring actions (what caring means to nurses and clients, and how it appears)

5. Caring consequences (outcomes of caring)

For the purposes of this exploration, the studies related to *caring conditions* and *consequences* will be summarized.

The category of *conditions* contains papers that explore variables affecting, enhancing, or inhibiting caring. "Nurse and patient experiences, backgrounds and/or personalities, society, organizations, health status and disease complications were all identified as influencing whether or not caring transpired."[26]

Patient-related conditions that influenced the establishment of a caring relationship were categorized as: communication, personality, health problems, care needs, and nurse-patient relationship. Findings suggested that patients who are grateful, who respond favorably, and who are honest about their feelings elicit favorable conditions for caring, whereas patients who are verbally abusive, unwilling to communicate, and resistive to support do not. Patients who are cheerful, accepting of their illnesses and vulnerability, alert, personable, outgoing, spirited and courageous, with a will to live, create conditions favorable to caring, whereas those who are combative, angry, hard to care for, in denial, and unattractive in personality may contribute to conditions in which caring is less likely to emerge. Findings also suggest that patients in pain, with uncertain outcomes, distressed, in crisis, and with psychosocial problems may facilitate a caring response in the nurse, whereas those with unpredictable problems may not. Based on these findings, it seems that patients with intense needs that can be met are more likely to experience caring than those with needs that may be intense but cannot be met. Finally, some qualities of the nurse-patient relationship, such as congruence in personalities and reciprocal interest, may favor caring, whereas disagreeable and argumentative relationships do not. In addition, the attractiveness of the patient may be related to conditions for caring.

The *nurse-related conditions* for caring are categorized as resources, constraints, and demands. Findings suggest that positive personal and professional resources such as past experiences, inner resources, education, and competence contribute to the likelihood that nurse caring will occur. Constraints to caring may be variables like tiredness, stress, feeling unappreciated or disrespected, witnessing death and suffering, or lack of knowledge and skills. Demands on the nurse that might inhibit caring are personal problems, the need to balance home and work, conflicts, and feeling overworked. Organization-related conditions that affect the occurrence of caring were categorized as personnel- or role-related, technology, administration, and work or practice conditions. A sense of community or teamwork seemed to be positive conditions for caring. Comfort with reliable technology and an administrative structure and staff that provide support, share governance, and promote communication were essential organizational conditions for caring. Working conditions that inhibit caring are lack of accountability for nurses, poor staffing, unreasonable workloads, and poor patient care.

Swanson's analysis of the literature on caring consequences has particular importance here. She reports that while some phenomenological investigations support Watson's[32] assertions that caring relationships lead to "betterment of both provider and recipient," there are few quantitative findings that support the outcomes of a caring relationship.[32] The lack of investigation of patient outcomes of caring is striking and lends support for this initiative. Two studies were identified as relevant exceptions to the lack of empirical work. Latham[33] examined the relationships among patient self-esteem, desire for information and control, nurse caring and the outcomes of appraisals, psychological distress, coping strategies, and effectiveness. "Forty percent of the overall variance in coping effectiveness was accounted for by the combined variables of supportive and sensitive caring, problem and emotion-focused coping and decreased psychological distress."[26] This correlational study lends support to caring as a contributing variable to the outcome of patient's coping effectiveness.

Duffy[34] studied the relationship between nurse caring, measured by the Caring Assessment Tool, and patient satisfaction, health status, length of stay, and health care costs. The only significant correlation $(r = 0.46, P < .001)$ was between caring and patient satisfaction.

Swanson summarized 30 qualitative studies conducted between 1986 and 1996 that described outcomes of caring and noncaring relationships. The studies' participants were nurses, patients and their families, students, family caregivers, and other health care providers. The outcomes of caring for the recipients of care were emotional and spiritual well-being (dignity, self-control, personhood), enhanced healing, and enhanced relationships. The consequences of noncaring were identified as feeling humiliated, frightened, out of control, desperate, helpless, alienated, and vulnerable. Significant nurse outcomes were a sense of personal and professional satisfaction and fulfillment. Consequences of noncaring for the nurse were feeling hardened, oblivious, depressed, frightened, and worn down.

Swanson's NIH-funded investigation of the effects of caring, measurement, and time on women's well-being during the first year subsequent to miscarrying is a notable contribution to the caring literature.[35] Using a randomized, controlled, Solomon 40–group experimental design, she determined that women randomized to 3-hour caring-based counseling sessions experienced less depressed, angry, and overall disturbed moods during the first year subsequent to miscarriage than controls who received no intervention.

In summary, the most extensive database on the concept most closely related to the healing relationship as it is defined in this Appendix is the literature on caring within the discipline of nursing. There is a wealth of qualitative data suggesting the importance of this relationship to the health and well-being of nurses and their patients and a dearth of outcomes studies to support these qualitative findings.

Developing Research on the Impact of the Healing Relationship

Given that there is virtually no previous research on the healing relationship as we have defined it and that research on the impact of caring, while congruent and inclusive of many elements of the healing relationship, remains primarily qualitative, it is our suggestion that exploratory, observational studies, triangulated with qualitative inquiry, provide the most appropriate starting point for discerning the impact of the healing relationship on selected outcomes. Observational designs, allowing for careful observation and measurement without manipulation of the variables, are consistent with the state of the science in the field; they could be used to address many of the questions for research that we have raised, and they are cost-effective.[36] Finally, they are consistent with nursing's theoretical frameworks.

Theoretical Frameworks for Investigating the Healing Relationship in Nursing

There are multiple conceptual frameworks in nursing within which the impact of the healing relationship has been or could be explored. Clearly the review of literature suggests that one of these is caring. The caring science framework developed by Jean Watson[2,37–40] has provided a foundation for research, practice, and education in nursing since 1979. Watson's framework posits the energetic nature of consciousness and that the caring consciousness emanates a quality of energy that potentiates healing. The caring/healing relationship preserves human dignity, wholeness, and integrity and is characterized by an authentic presencing and choice. Watson articulates the transpersonal nature of the healing relationship when she defines an instance of it as a "caring moment"[3] in which the soul of the nurse and the soul of the patient come into relationship and are both changed by the interaction.

Other nurse theorists, both before and after Watson, also have explicated the concept of caring as central to nursing. For example, through three separate phenomenological investigations of women experiencing perinatal loss, Swanson developed a middle-range theory of caring, which she tested through the randomized study mentioned above.[35] Swanson[41,42] defines caring as "a nurturing way of relating to a valued other towards whom one feels a personal sense of commitment and responsibility." She has defined five processes by which caring is enacted:

1. *Knowing* means striving to understand an event as it has meaning in the life of the other

2. *Being with* is being emotionally present

3. *Doing for* is doing what the other would do for himself or herself if it were at all possible

4. *Enabling* is facilitating the other's passage through life events and transitions by providing information, validation, and support

5. *Maintaining belief* is sustaining faith in the capacity of the other to get through events or transitions and face a future with meaning

In the 1999 paper on the state of caring science reviewed above,[41] Swanson provided evidence from 67 separate qualitative investigations of caring actions that suggest her characterization of the caring relationship may be generalizable beyond the perinatal setting.

Newman's framework offers another related perspective within which the healing relationship can be studied. Newman, Sime, and Corcoran-Perry identify the need for nursing practice and research to move from a particularistic or deterministic paradigm to a unitary or transformative paradigm.[43] Within the unitary or transformative perspective, they suggest, "a phenomenon is viewed as a unitary, self-organizing field embedded in a larger self-organizing field. Change is unidirectional and unpredictable as systems move through stages of organization and disorganization to more complex organization. Knowledge is personal, involves pattern recognition and is a function of both the viewer and the phenomenon viewed."[43] Within this framework, the healing relationship would be explored as a whole system, not as a sum of the parts.

Smith's[44] analysis of the caring literature through a unitary lens resulted in the elaboration of five constituents of caring:

1. Manifesting intention
2. Appreciating pattern
3. Attuning to dynamic flow
4. Experiencing the infinite
5. Inviting creative emergence

These elements may contribute to the explication of the healing relationship as defined earlier in this paper.

Based on a classic qualitative study, Halldorsdottir[45] developed a classification of nurse-patient relationships that forms a continuum from uncaring to caring and to which we could add from nonhealing to healing, as follows:

- Type 1 is biocidic or life-destroying (toxic, leading to anger, despair, and decreased well-being)
- Type 2 is biostatic or life-restraining (cold or treated as a nuisance)
- Type 3 is biopassive or life-neutral (apathetic or detached)
- Type 4 is bioactive or life-sustaining (classic nurse-patient relationship as kind, concerned, and benevolent)
- Type 5 is biogenic or life-giving.

"This [biogenic] mode involves loving benevolence, responsiveness, generosity, mercy and compassion. A truly life-giving presence offers the other interconnectedness and fosters spiritual freedom. It involves being open to persons and giving life to the very heart of man as person, creating a relationship of openness and receptivity yet always keeping a creative distance of respect and compassion. The truly life-giving or biogenic presence restores well being and human dignity. It is a transforming personal presence that deeply changes one. For the recipient there is experienced an inrush of compassion, often like a current."[45]

The biogenic relationship, we would propose, is the healing relationship and closely parallels Watson's "caring moment."[3]

Finally, there is the framework of Florence Nightingale, who suggested that it is only nature that ultimately cures (heals) and that the role of the nurse is "to put the patient in the best condition for nature to act upon him."[4] It seems reasonable to assume that the probable mechanism for the impact of the healing relationship in the health care encounter is exactly this: the healing relationship puts the person in the best condition for nature to act on him or her. The human-to-human relationship has the capacity to mediate a host of psychophysiological processes for better or for worse. Miller and colleagues[46] offer a related discussion." Insofar as anxiety, stress, depression, and fear are negative influences on health, then clinician-patient relationships that create these states of body-mind-spirit might be thought of as 'unhealing'" relationships or, in Halldorsdottir's model, biocidal. The biogenic or healing relationship assists in creating the conditions by which the innate tendency toward the emergence of healing is facilitated and enhanced in terms of renewal, order, increased coherence, and transformation—the Haelan effect in Quinn's[47-50] framework. Here, the enormous literature in psychoneuroimmunology, social support, love, and systems and chaos theories can be useful. For example, social support has been shown to affect health status, as has love. The healing relationship might be viewed as a type of critical social support and as a particular kind of love offered in moments of intense disequilibrium and vulnerability. It is, perhaps, the added energy in the system that allows the patient to emerge out of the chaos into a higher order—in other words, healing.

Issues in the Design of Studies on the Healing Relationship in Clinical Nursing Practice

1. *Research methods need to reflect the nature of the healing relationship.*

It seems a fair assessment of the literature related to the healing relationship to say that it is particularistic rather than unitary. That is, most studies examined one or more personal characteristics of clinicians, such as empathy, listening behaviors, or communication styles, and then correlated various types of scores on these measures with one or more patient outcomes, usually patient satisfaction, as noted above.

Within the caring/healing frameworks of Watson,[2,37-40] Swanson,[41-42] and others, the unitary-transformative paradigm developed by Newman, Sime, and Corcoran-Perry,[43] and the modes of relationship described by Halldorsdottir,[45] it would seem that the healing relationship is better understood as being more than and different from the sum of its parts. As a living system, adaptive and chaotic, it is nonlinear and acausal. This is also the consensus reached among researchers gathered at the International Workshop on Research Methods for the Investigation of Complementary and Alternative Medicine Whole Systems, which took place in October 2002 in Vancouver, British Columbia.

While there may be correlates of the presence of the healing relationship, such as warmth, compassion, caring behaviors, empathy, and the rest, none of these, especially when isolated from the others, can tell us about the whole, which is a living process occurring within and between two whole, unitary human beings. Furthermore, prescriptive approaches may, in fact, produce the opposite of a healing relationship, creating a sort of script that can inoculate the clinician against the emergence of authentic presence that has been identified throughout the literature as a critical element.

Thus, one major challenge to developing research protocols that can assess the impact of the healing relationship is designing studies that can assess the healing relationship as a whole system. At this juncture, it seems reasonable to suggest that exploratory, observational study designs are most appropriate as approaches to provide initial assessments of associations between some measure of the healing relationship and some specified outcomes. Several principles need to guide the selection of research designs within the broad category of descriptive, observational studies.

A. Study of both members of the healing relationship. Such an approach is consistent with a whole systems approach and with nursing's unitary paradigm, allowing for the possibility of actually seeing patterns of the whole system that is the relationship rather than limiting the exploration to one part or the other. Because the healing relationship involves (at least) two individuals engaged in a mutual, simultaneous process, it is conceptually incomplete to limit the focus of research on the impact of the healing relationship to only the patient, client, or healee. Clearly, there is a need to understand the experiences of both the healer and healee and their contributions to the dynamic they co-create. Moreover, the health/well-being of those caring is as legitimate a concern for research on the impact of the healing relationship as that of the ones cared for. The nursing literature is rich in its testimony to the importance of being able to engage in meaningful relationships with patients as a source of satisfaction, joy, and healing for nurses as well as the costs to nurses when such relationship is prevented.

Quinn conducted a descriptive pilot study of both the practitioners and recipients of Therapeutic Touch within this framework and examined psychological and immunological outcomes in both.[51] Of interest to the exploration of the relationship between healer and healee is her finding that each dyad manifested a pattern of time perception and distortion that varied during a series of 7 treatments delivered over 10 days. When one member of the dyad overestimated the length of a treatment, so did the other member. If one underestimated, the other underestimated. Different patterns; i.e., overestimating or underestimating, occurred for each treatment session, but the dyad, in three out of the four dyads studied, always varied together. Inasmuch as the experience of time passing is an index of state of consciousness, it is possible that what was being observed was a correlate of authentic presence and shared consciousness within the healing relationship.

B. *Multiple ways of knowing are required to explore the full range of multidimensional questions raised about the healing relationship.* Carper's[52] work in nursing provides one such framework that identifies the following four patterns of knowing:

1. Empirical (five-sense data; the science of nursing)

2. Esthetic (taking in the whole; perception; the art of nursing, including empathic acquaintance)

3. Personal (an intuitive or subjective way of knowing; relational; encountering and actualizing the concrete, individual self)

4. Ethical (the moral component; matters of obligation; the way things ought to be)

An integral model for research on the healing relationship based on Wilber and Walsh's four quadrants of existence[53] is consistent with nursing's caring science framework (see Figure A1-1). In this model, the quadrants represent a summary of a data search across various developmental and evolutionary fields, including over 200 developmental sequences recognized by various branches of knowledge ranging from stellar physics to molecular biology, from anthropology to linguistics, from developmental psychology to ethical orientations, from cultural hermeneu-

Figure A1-1

An Integral Model for Research on the Healing Relationship

	INTERIOR	EXTERIOR
COLLECTIVE	Subjective *As known / experienced / lived by individual nurse and patient:* • Phenomenological inquiry • Narrative/story • Participant/observer • Others	Objective *As measured outcomes related to nurse and patient:* • Nurse and patient satisfaction • Quality of life, global health, spiritual well-being • Physiological or environmental monitoring during nurse-patient encounters • Physiological monitoring during postencounter interviews • Others
INDIVIDUAL	Intersubjective *As known between nurse and patient:* • Assessment of common themes/ experiences in narratives • Shared interviews • Nurse-patient dialogue • Others	Interobjective *As measured outcomes related to systems:* • Staff satisfaction • Staff turnover • System or unit-wide patient satisfaction • Comparisons between different hospitals in same system • Others

Adapted with permission from Wilber K, Walsh R. An integral approach to consciousness research. In Velmans M. *Investigating Phenomenal Consciousness: New Methodologies and Maps*. Philadelphia: John Benjamins, 2000.

tics to contemplative endeavors. They include both Eastern and Western disciplines as well as premodern, modern, and postmodern sources.[52]

The two quadrants on the right represent the individual (upper-right quadrant) and the collective (lower-right quadrant) dimensions that can be known through the senses or their extensions. Empirical knowing is a product of research originating in one of these two quadrants. They are objective and interobjective, and exterior. The two quadrants on the left are the interior dimensions of the individual (upper-left quadrant) and the collective (lower-left quadrant).

Fully exploring the impact of the healing relationship in nursing will mean that research questions and methods will need to address all the quadrants as follows:

❄ Questions related to the lived experience of the healing relationship for the patient and the clinician as individuals would be upper-left quadrant questions and would require one or more types of qualitative inquiry.

❄ Questions related to the shared experience of the healing relationship would be lower-left quadrant questions, requiring interview data or correlational approaches.

❄ Questions related to the impact of the healing relationship on observable, measurable outcomes are upper-right quadrant questions, which lend themselves to quantitative methods and designs.

❄ Questions related to how the healing relationship is manifested in and impacts on systems of health care would be lower-right quadrant questions. Health services research designs might be employed here.

It is our recommendation that research in this new area begin with questions from the upper-right quadrant, which can be addressed through an observational outcomes design, enriched by subjective data that could address the upper-left quadrant perspective; i.e., the lived experience of the healing relationship in both nurses and patients. Therefore, research should include both qualitative, self-report measures and quantitative, observable, third-person measures. Such triangulated designs have a long history in nursing.

2. *Measurement tools need to be consistent with the theoretical framework for the study and the conceptual definitions of both independent and dependent variables.*

A. *Measurement related to healing as an outcome (the dependent variable).* Measurement of healing, including measures that can indicate healing in the absence of curing, healing as renewal, transformation, or wholeness, requires tools that are consistent with a whole systems approach. Because there are few extant tools that assess healing as a whole as it is defined here, tool development is a critical activity at this stage of the discipline.

There are some tools that, although they do not specifically measure healing as a whole, can indicate outcomes that could certainly be seen as aspects of healing and therefore be useful to link to the healing relationship. Whatever tools are chosen or developed, a rationale should be provided that carefully establishes the validity of the measure relative to the construct of healing as it is being defined here; that is, as more than and different from the cure of physical disease. Table A1-1 summarizes some of these tools. Of particular note is the McGill Quality of Life Questionnaire[54–57] with its inclusion of an existential domain in addition to the physical and psychological domains of being. This tool has well-established reliability and validity.

In addition, it is appropriate, particularly because this is a new field of inquiry, to include one or more measures that are typically used in the particular population being studied to measure health-related outcomes so that the contribution of the healing relationships to these standard measures might be assessed.

Finally, global measures with established reliability and validity that are typically used across populations to assess health-related outcomes, such as patient satisfaction with nursing care, should be included.[74] The data from such inquiry may ground the findings of the study in a language familiar to practitioners and decision-makers across the levels of health care administration and management.

Whatever outcome measures are chosen should be presented with a clear rationale that specifies the following:

1. How they are consistent with the conceptual or theoretical framework for the study, or if they are not consistent, why their use is appropriate

2. Protocols for tool development, including testing for validity and reliability

3. The patient-centered focus of the measure; that is, if and why this measure matters to patients and justifies the use of their time and energy to provide the data

B. Measurement related to the caring/healing relationship (the independent or process variable). There are no instruments available that can adequately operationalize the occurrence of the whole of the healing relationship. Extant tools for measuring caring might be useful. Watson's 2002 compendium[75] of instruments for assessing and measuring caring includes tools that measure quality of care, patient and nurse perceptions of caring, caring behaviors, caring abilities, and caring efficacy. These 21 instruments, developed by a variety of researchers, can be useful in measuring the extent to which a caring/healing relationship exists and in this way can contribute to

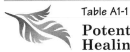

Table A1-1

Potential Instruments to Measure Outcomes of Healing Relationships in Adult Populations

INSTRUMENT NAME (ABBREVIATION)	AUTHORS	DESCRIPTION	LANGUAGE	NUMBER OF ITEMS
General Well-Being Schedule (GWB)	Dupuy[58]	Measures psychological well-being through representations of subjective well-being or distress	English, possibly other translations	22
Life Orientation Test (LOT)	Scheier, Carver[59]	Measures dispositional optimism or the expectancy to experience positive outcomes	English, possibly other translations	12
Long-Term Quality of Life (LTQL)	Wyatt, Kurtz, Friedman, Given, Given[60]	Measures quality of life for long-term female cancer survivors; includes spiritual and philosophical views of life	English	34
McGill Quality of Life Questionnaire (MQOL)	Cohen, Mount[61]	Measures quality of life in those with advanced cancer	English	17
Multidimensional Quality of Life Scale (MQOLS)	Padilla, Mishel, Grant[62]	Adapted from Padilla's earlier QLI instrument for people with cancer; measures quality of life in domains of psychological, physical well-being, symptom control, finances	English	27
Psychological General Well-Being (PGWB)	Dupuy[58]	Self-reports of affective states reflecting subjective well-being or distress	More than 25 languages	22
Purpose in Life Test (PIL)	Crumbaugh, Maholick[63]	Assesses purpose in life based on Frank's theory of meaning	English, possibly other translations	20

(continued)

Table A1-1 *(Continued)*

Potential Instruments to Measure Outcomes of Healing Relationships in Adult Populations

INSTRUMENT NAME (ABBREVIATION)	AUTHORS	DESCRIPTION	LANGUAGE	NUMBER OF ITEMS
Quality of Life Index (QLI)	Ferrans, Powers[64]	Measures quality of life in terms of satisfaction with life	12 languages, including English, French, Spanish, Japanese, Russian, and Swedish	66
Quality of Life Scale (QOLS)	Flanagan,[65] modified by Burkhardt et al[66]	Measures quality of life for those with chronic illness	12 languages including English, German, Swedish, Hebrew, Mandarin Chinese, Danish	16
Schedule for the Evaluation of Individual Quality of Life (SElQoL)	O'Boyle,[67] McGee,[68] Hickey, Joyce, Browne, O'Malley, Hillbrunner	Assesses quality of life from an individual	English	30
Self-Transcendence Scale (STS)	Reed[69]	Assesses intrapersonal, interpersonal, and temporal experiences that reflect expanded boundaries of self	English, possibly other translations	30
Sense of Coherence Scale (SOC-29)	Antonovsky[70]	Measures life's comprehensibility, manageability, and meaningfulness	English, possibly other translations	29
Spiritual Well-Being Index (SWB)	Paloutzian and Ellison[71]	Measures spiritual well-being and existential well-being	English, possibly other translations	20

(continued)

Table A1-1 *(Continued)*

Potential Instruments to Measure Outcomes of Healing Relationships in Adult Populations

INSTRUMENT NAME (ABBREVIATION)	AUTHORS	DESCRIPTION	LANGUAGE	NUMBER OF ITEMS
Spiritual Perspective Scale (SPS)	Reed[72]	Measures saliency of spirituality, the extent that spirituality permeates their lives, and extent of engagement in spiritual interactions	English, possibly other translations	10
WHO Quality of Life (WHOQOL)*	WHO Quality of Life Group[73]	Assesses individual perceptions of the quality of their lives	Available in more than 30 translations	100
WHO Quality of Life Brief (WHOQOL-BREF)	WHO Quality of Life Group[73]	Assesses individual perceptions of the quality of their lives	Available in more than 30 translations	26

*WHO: World Health Organization

operationalizing the independent variable in the development of impact studies on the healing relationship.

In our review of the literature, we found that the schema presented by Halldorsdottir[45] could quite easily lend itself to the development of a rating instrument for use by both patients and nurses. Individual nurse-patient relationships could be rated from "biocidic" to "biogenic" by patients and nurses, and these scores could be correlated with selected outcome measures related to healing in patients and satisfaction and burnout in nurses. This Appendix comprises a draft for such a tool, which draws its terms from the extant literature on caring. Scores on this tool also could provide the indication for a qualitative interview with both nurses and patients. If, for example, a particular nurse-patient relationship was scored as biogenic by one or the other member of the dyad, it would be important to collect additional information about what the experience was, what it meant to the reporting person(s), and how the person(s) perceived the effect of the experience. This triangulated design would explore the impact of the healing relationship through questions and methods associated with the upper-right quadrant, the upper-left quadrant, and the lower-left quadrant in the model for integrative research presented earlier.

C. *Emergent novel measures.* One approach to assessing the quality of the nurse-patient relationship for its healing versus nonhealing impact is by asking patients about their experience of the relationship as suggested above. One might consider that, just as in assessing pain, it is now a given that "pain is what the patient says it is"; healing and the healing relationship might be similarly determined.

It also may be possible to observe physiological processes as a way to assess nurse-patient relationships. Physiological responses of patients to particular nurses can be measured after the relationship has concluded as a way of obtaining the following information:

❁ Concurrent validity with paper and pencil scales

❁ Unconscious responses

❁ Initial indicators of the physiological correlates of healing

❁ Initial indicators of both healing and nonhealing relationships

For example, Halldorsdottir describes the biocidic relationship as one in which the patient is actually harmed by the practitioner through manipulation, coercion, abuse, humiliation, or other forms of physical, mental, emotional, or spiritual violence. She says "it involves the transference of negative energy or darkness to the other . . . the harm done depending on the other's strength to endure."[45] Are there physiological correlates to this relationship that might be accessible to measurement? Similarly, are there correlates of the relationship that are biogenic? Such measures might contribute to a model that more fully explains what part the provider-patient relationship plays in "putting the patient in the best condition for nature to act upon him"[4] by telling us something about the inner environment that is created through the relationship.

One way to collect these data would be to use a computer with a simple biofeedback measurement capacity. Patients could be physiologically monitored while they viewed, serially and with appropriate baseline times between, pictures of the various nurses with whom they had relationships during the period being studied. Patients also would complete outcomes questionnaires about each of these nurses on the computer. Responses to the questionnaire assessing a patient's perception of the healing nature of the relationship could be correlated with physiological data about the same nurse and with the healing outcome measures for a broad overview of the impact of the healing relationship.

166

3. *Preservation of the nature of the healing relationship while trying to study it.*

Observational studies and naturalistic inquiry, unlike clinical trials, do not attempt to manipulate or change the independent variable. These types of study can minimize but not resolve the issue of inadvertently affecting the healing relationship. One needs to acknowledge that by the very process of observing (querying, measuring) the relationship, the relationship is changed. Researchers need to address this problem in their designs and be explicit in their decisions regarding how to address these issues. Confounding variables need to be addressed through the design of the research study.

Clinical research in this area is complicated by the vast number of parameters that are outside of the control of the healing dyad. Issues such as staffing, mandatory overtime, organizational structures, discharge or transfer decisions, and other concerns may impact on the nurses' opportunity and capacity to form healing relationships with their patients as well as on the patients' health-related outcomes. Research designs need to acknowledge these variables and describe steps taken to mitigate their impact.

Further Considerations in Designing the Research

1. *Participants*

An observational study on the impact of the healing relationship in clinical nursing practice could take place in virtually any setting and with any population of patients with whom nurses interact. For example, any hospital could select one of its units, say the oncology unit, to explore this question. The research question would be: What is the impact of the healing relationship on (selected) outcomes of hospitalized oncology patients and on their nurses?

Another valuable approach would be to explore this question with several different populations, or across different units in the same hospital, or across similar units in different hospitals, thus illuminating the lower-right quadrant perspective. For example, would patients in hospitals that espouse relationship-centered care experience the nurse-patient relationship as more healing than patients in hospitals without such an emphasis? Would selected outcomes vary across these settings?

Whatever participants are selected, the rationale related to the questions for study, as well as eligibility criteria and methods for recruitment, should be specified.

2. *Specific objectives and hypotheses*

Specific objectives should be presented in the form of research questions, as in the following example: Is there an association between

Draft of a Nurse-Patient Relationship Questionnaire

Jane Doe, RN

1. Choose one:
   - ☐ This nurse took care of me.
   - ☐ This nurse did not take care of me.

Jane Doe, RN

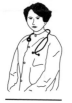

2. Looking at this picture makes me feel (CHOOSE ONE):
   - ☐ Cold and disgusted; Sad
   - ☐ Nothing
   - ☐ Warm and peaceful; Deeply moved

Jane Doe, RN

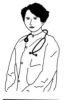

3. How CONNECTED to this nurse did you feel (CHOOSE ONE):
   - ☐ Very unconnected
   - ☐ Somewhat unconnected
   - ☐ Neither connected nor unconnected
   - ☐ Somewhat connected
   - ☐ Very connected

Jane Doe, RN

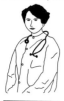

4. In my relationship with this nurse, I felt that my DIGNITY was (CHOOSE ONE):
   - ☐ Destroyed
   - ☐ Hurt
   - ☐ Unaffected
   - ☐ Preserved
   - ☐ Enhanced

Jane Doe, RN

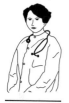

5. In my relationship with this nurse, I felt that my PHYSICAL WELL-BEING was (CHOOSE ONE):
   - ☐ Destroyed
   - ☐ Hurt
   - ☐ Unaffected
   - ☐ Preserved
   - ☐ Enhanced

(continued)

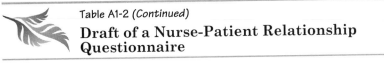

Draft of a Nurse-Patient Relationship Questionnaire

Jane Doe, RN

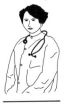

6. In my relationship with this nurse, I felt that my EMOTIONAL WELL-BEING was (CHOOSE ONE):
   - ☐ Destroyed
   - ☐ Hurt
   - ☐ Unaffected
   - ☐ Preserved
   - ☐ Enhanced

Jane Doe, RN

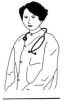

7. In my relationship with this nurse, I felt that my SPIRITUAL WELL-BEING was (CHOOSE ONE):
   - ☐ Destroyed
   - ☐ Hurt
   - ☐ Unaffected
   - ☐ Preserved
   - ☐ Enhanced

Jane Doe, RN

8. In my relationship with this nurse, I felt that my HEALING was (CHOOSE ONE):
   - ☐ Destroyed
   - ☐ Hurt
   - ☐ Unaffected
   - ☐ Preserved
   - ☐ Enhanced

Jane Doe, RN

9. In my relationship with this nurse, I felt that my SENSE OF WHOLENESS was (CHOOSE ONE):
   - ☐ Destroyed.
   - ☐ Hurt
   - ☐ Unaffected
   - ☐ Preserved
   - ☐ Enhanced

Jane Doe, RN

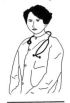

10. In my relationship with this nurse, I felt that my SENSE OF SAFETY was (CHOOSE ONE):
    - ☐ Destroyed
    - ☐ Hurt
    - ☐ Unaffected
    - ☐ Preserved
    - ☐ Enhanced

(continued)

Table A1-2 *(Continued)*

Draft of a Nurse-Patient Relationship Questionnaire

Jane Doe, RN

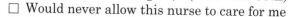

11. If I were hospitalized again, I (CHOOSE ONE):
    ☐ Would never allow this nurse to care for me
    ☐ Would not like this nurse to care for me
    ☐ Would not care if this nurse cared for me or not
    ☐ Would want this nurse to care for me
    ☐ Would be thrilled to have this nurse care for me

Jane Doe, RN

12. Words I would use to describe this nurse are (write in as few/many as you like):

how oncology patients rate the healing quality of their relationships with nursing staff and patient satisfaction with nursing care following discharge? Hypotheses that include the specific data to be collected should be specified as the basis for data analysis. For example, from the research question/objective above, a testable hypothesis would be the following: At 48 hours postdischarge, oncology patients who rate at least one nurse-patient relationship as healing on the healing-relationship scale have higher scores on the patient-satisfaction-with-nursing-care questionnaire than patients who do not rate any nurse-patient relationship as healing.

3. *Sample size*

The sample size for the study should be specified, along with a discussion of how the number was determined. Recognizing that ideal sample sizes are not always possible to obtain in clinical nursing settings, the sample should be large enough to have sufficient power to detect a statistically significant association between the independent and dependent variables if, in fact, an association exists.

4. *Statistical methods*

Specific methods for analyzing the data should be presented for each hypothesis, along with a rationale for the appropriateness of their

Checklist Quality Guidelines for Developing a Research Protocol to Assess Impact of Healing Relationship in Clinical Nursing Practice

PROTOCOL SECTION	CRITERIA
Title and abstract	The title clearly identifies the study as an observational or impact study focused not on efficacy but on assessment of the impact of the healing relationship in clinical nursing practice. The term *healing relationship* appears in the title so that the healing relationship as field of study begins to become more widely recognized and so that the study may be easily located by future researchers. The abstract is structured so that the objective(s), design, setting, participants, and main outcome measures are easily identified.
Scientific background and explanation of rationale	Research on this topic expands one or more of the rationales offered in this paper, or another rationale is offered to justify the significance of the study. Following this discussion, a rationale is offered for the particular approach taken in the study, based on extant literature and related theories, where appropriate. Specific questions about the healing relationship, which the study will help to answer, are presented in either question form or as objectives or aims. The list of 20 questions provided earlier in this chapter is not exhaustive but may assist researchers in focusing their inquiry. Independent and dependent variables are defined, and rationales are provided for their selection, grounded in extant nursing and related theoretical frameworks.
Methods	A rationale is provided for the methods and design chosen, based on theoretical rationale and questions for study.

(continued)

Checklist Quality Guidelines for Developing a Research Protocol to Assess Impact of Healing Relationship in Clinical Nursing Practice

Research methods need to reflect the nature of the healing relationship.	• The study includes both members of the healing relationship: nurses and patients. • Multiple ways of knowing are used: both quantitative and qualitative data are collected.
Measurement tools need to be consistent with the theoretical framework for the study and the conceptual definitions of both independent and dependent variables.	• Measurement tools are fully described, and a rationale for their use is presented. • Any tools developed are described, including a rationale and any measures taken to establish validity and reliability.
Preservation of the healing relationship while trying to study it	The study includes a discussion of issues related to preserving the healing relationship; measures taken to minimize disturbance are described.
Confounding variables need to be addressed through the design of the research study	Confounding variables particular to the setting and population being studied are identified; measures taken to mitigate their effects are described.
Participants	Eligibility criteria and a rationale for selecting nurse and patient participants are provided; the setting(s) for data collection are described.
Specific objectives and hypotheses	Specific objectives are presented in the form of research questions. Where appropriate, hypotheses that include the specific data to be collected are specified as the basis for data analysis.

(continued)

Table A1-3 *(Continued)*

Checklist Quality Guidelines for Developing a Research Protocol to Assess Impact of Healing Relationship in Clinical Nursing Practice

Sample size	The sample size for the study is specified, along with a discussion of how the number was determined and how participants will be recruited.
Statistical methods	Specific methods for analyzing the data are presented for each hypothesis, with a rationale for the appropriateness of the methods' use. If additional qualitative data are needed, then methods for collecting and analyzing these data and ensuring rigor also are specified.

use. If there is to be additional analysis, for example, to include qualitative data derived from interviews, then methods for collecting and analyzing these data and ensuring rigor also should be specified.

References

1. Dossey, L. (2003). Samueli conference on definitions and standards in healing research: working definitions and terms. *Alternative Therapies in Health and Medicine, 9*(Suppl. 3), 13A–15A.
2. American Nurses Association. (1980, 1995). *Nursing's Social Policy Statement.* Washington, DC: American Nurses Publishing.
3. Watson, J. (1985). *Nursing: The philosophy and science of caring.* Boulder, CO: University of Colorado Press.
4. Nightingale, F. (1969). *Notes on nursing: What it is and what it is not.* New York: Dover Press.
5. Quinn, J.F. (2002). Revisioning the nursing shortage: A call to caring for healing the healthcare system. *Frontiers of Health Services Management, 19*(2):3–21.
6. Gellert-Ross, J.C. (1997) Healing hearts: A heuristic study of the experience of women in myriad healing professions. *Dissertation Abstracts International A.* Ann Arbor, MI: University Microfilms International, *57,*11A.
7. Montgomery, C. (1994). The caring/healing relationship of maintaining authentic caring. In J. Watson (Ed.), *Applying the art and science of human caring* (pp 39–45). New York: National League for Nursing.
8. Pellegrino, E. (1987). Toward a reconstruction of medical morality. *Journal of Medical Humanities and Bioethics, 8*(1):7–18.
9. Druss, R. (2000). *Listening to patients: Relearning the art of healing in psychotherapy.* New York: Oxford University Press.

10. Dacher, E. (1999). Loving openness and the healing relationship. *Advances in Mind-Body Medicine, 15*(1):24–27.

11. Dirschel, K.M. (1998). Nursing care of the stroke patient: the essence of healing. In W. Sife (Ed.). *After stroke: Enhancing quality of life. Loss, grief and care* (pp71–78). Binghamton, NY: Haworth Press.

12. Aylor, R. (1993). The healing relationship. *Revolution, 3*(4):18–19.

13. Merkle, W.F. (1993). Bringing empathic awareness beyond the self: An interdisciplinary approach to the healing relationship. *Dissertation Abstracts International A.* Ann Arbor, MI: University Microfilms International, *53,*12A.

14. Appelbaum, S.A. (1988). Psychoanalytic therapy: A subset of healing. *Psychotherapy, 25*(2):201–208.

15. Saba, G., & Fink, D.L. (1985). Systems medicine and systems therapy: A call to a natural collaboration. *Journal of Strategic Systems Therapy, 4*(2):15–31.

16. Burton, A. (1979). The mentoring factor in the therapeutic relationship. *Psychoanalytic Revue, 66*(4):507–517.

17. Friedman, M. (1975). Healing through meeting: A dialogical approach to psychotherapy. Part 1. *American Journal of Psychoanalysis, 35*(3):255–267.

18. Horvath, A.O., & Symonds, B.D. (1991) Relation between working alliance and outcome in psychotherapy: A meta-analysis. *Journal of Counseling Psychology 38*(2):139–149.

19. Strupp, H.H., & Hadley, S.W. (1979). Specific vs nonspecific factors in psychotherapy. A controlled study of outcome. *Archives of General Psychiatry 36*(10):1125–1136.

20. Orlinsky, D.E., & Howard K.I.L. (1985). Therapy process and outcome. In S. Garfield, & A. Bergin (Eds.). *Handbook of psychotherapy and behavior change* (pp 311–381). New York: John Wiley & Sons.

21. Luborsky, L., Crits-Cristoph, P., Mclellan, A.T., et al. (1986). Do therapists vary much in their success? Findings from four outcome studies. *American Journal of Orthopsychiatry, 56*(4):501–512.

22. Herman, K. (1993). Reassessing predictors of therapist competence. *J Couns Dev, 72*(5):29–32.

23. Martin, D.J., Garske, J.P., & Davis, K.M. (2000). Relation of the therapeutic alliance with outcome and other variables: A meta-analytic review. *J Consult Clin Psychol, 68*(3):438–450.

24. Fanning, J.J. (1998). Relationships between healers' spirituality and their beliefs about healing. *Dissertation Abstracts International B.* Ann Arbor, MI: University Microfilms International *59,* 6B.

25. Little, P., Williamson, I., Warner, G., Moore, M., Gould, C., Ferrier, K., & Payne, S. (2001). Observational study of effect of patient centeredness and positive approach on outcomes of general practice consultations. *British Medical Journal, 323*(7318):908–911.

26. Stewart, M., Brown, J.B., Donner, A., McWhinney, I.R., Oates, J., Weston, W., & Jordan, J. (2000). The impact of patient-centered care on outcomes. *Journal of Family Practice, 49*(9):796–804.

27. Kaplan, S.H., Greenfield, S., & Ware, J.E. Jr. (1989). Assessing the effects of physician-patient interactions on the outcomes of chronic disease. *Medical Care, 27*(Suppl 3): S110–S127.

28. Adams, R.J., Smith, B.J., & Ruffin, R.E. (2001). Impact of physician's participatory style in asthma outcomes and patient satisfaction. *Annals of Allergy, Asthma, and Immunology, 86*(3):263–271.

29. Jackson, J.I., & Kroenke, K. (2001). The effect of unmet expectations among adults

presenting with physical symptoms. *Annals of Internal Medicine, 134*(Suppl 9, Pt 2):889–897.

30. Mead N., & Bower P. (2000). Patient-centeredness: a conceptual framework and review of the empirical literature. *Social Science and Medicine, 51*(7):1087–1110.

31. Swanson, K: (1999). What is known about caring in nursing science: A literary meta-analysis. In A.S. Hinshaw, S. Feetham, & J. Shaver (Eds.). *Handbook of clinical nursing research* (pp. 31–60). Thousand Oaks, CA: Sage.

32. Watson, M.J. (1988). *Nursing: Human science and human care.* New York: National League for Nursing.

33. Latham, C.P. (1996). Predictors of patient outcomes following interaction with nurses. *Western Journal of Nursing Research, 18*(5):548–564.

34. Duffy, J.R. (1992). Impact of nurse caring on patient outcomes. In D.A. Gaut (Ed.). *The Presence of caring in nursing* (pp. 365-377). New York: National League for Nursing.

35. Swanson, K.M. (1999). Effects of caring, measurement and time on miscarriage impact and women's well being. *Nursing Research 48*(6):288–298.

36. Walach, H., Jonas, W.B., & Lewith, G. (2002). The role of outcomes research in evaluating complementary and alternative medicine. In *Clinical research in complementary therapies: Principles, problems and solutions* (pp. 29–45). Edinburgh, Scotland: Churchill Livingstone.

37. Watson, J. (1999). *Postmodern nursing and beyond.* Edinburgh, Scotland: Churchill Livingstone/WB Saunders.

38. Watson, J. (1998). Nightingale and the enduring legacy of transpersonal human caring. *Journal of Holistic Nursing, 16*(2):292–294.

39. Watson, J. (1995). Nursing's caring-healing model as exemplar for alternative medicine. *Alternative Therapies in Health and Medicine, 1*(3):64–69.

40. Watson, J., & Smith, M.C. (2002). Caring science and the science of unitary human beings: A trans-theoretical discourse for nursing knowledge development. *Journal of Advanced Nursing, 37*(5);452–461.

41. Swanson, K. (1991). Empirical development of a middle-range theory of caring. *Nursing Research, 40*(3):161–166.

42. Swanson, K. (1993). Nursing as informed caring for the well-being of others. *Image: The Journal of Nursing Scholarship, 25*(4):352–357.

43. Newman, M.A., Sime, A.M., & Corcoran-Perry, S.A. (1991). The focus of the discipline of nursing. *Advanced Nursing Science, 14*(1):1–6.

44. Smith, M. (1992). Caring and the science of unitary human beings. *Advanced Nursing Science, 21*(4):14–28.

45. Halldorsdottir, S. (1991). Five basic modes of being with another. In D.A. Gaut, & M. Leininger (Eds.). *Caring: The compassionate healer.* New York: National League for Nursing.

46. Miller, W.L., Crabtree, B.F., Duffy, M.B., Epstein, R.M., & Stange, K.C. (2003). Research guidelines for assessing the impact of the healing relationship in clinical medicine. *Alternative Therapies in Health and Medicine, 9*(Suppl 3):85A–101A.

47. Quinn, J.F. (1989). On healing, wholeness and the Haelan effect. *Nursing and Health Care, 10*(10);553–556.

48. Quinn, J.F. (1992). Holding sacred space: The nurse as healing environment. *Holistic Nursing Practice, 6*(4):26–35.

49. Quinn, J.F. (1997). Healing: A model for an integrative health care system. *Advanced Practice Nursing Quarterly, 3*(1):1–7.

50. Quinn, J.F. (2000). Transpersonal human caring and healing. In B. Dossey (Ed.). *Holistic nursing: A handbook for practice* (3rd ed). Gaithersburg, MD: Aspen.

51. Quinn, J.F. (1993). Psychoimmunologic effects of therapeutic touch on practitioners

and recently bereaved recipients: A pilot study. *Advanced Nursing Science, 15*(4):13–26.

52. Carper, B. (1978). Fundamental patterns of knowing in nursing. *Advanced Nursing Science, 1*(1):13–23.
53. Wilber, K., & Walsh, R. (2000). An integral approach to consciousness research. In M. Velmans (Ed.). *Investigating phenomenal consciousness: New methodologies and maps.* Philadelphia: John Benjamins.
54. Cohen, S.R., Mount, B.M., Tomas, J.J., & Mount, L.F. (1996). Existential well-being is an important determinant of quality of life. Evidence from the McGill Quality of Life Questionnaire. *Cancer, 77*(3):576–586.
55. Cohen, S.R., Mount, B.M., Bruera, E., Provost, M., Rowe, J., & Tong, K. (1997). Validity of the McGill Quality of Life Questionnaire in the palliative care setting: A multi-centre Canadian study demonstrating the importance of the existential domain. *Palliative Medicine, 11*(1):3–0.
56. Cohen, S.R., & Mount, B. M. (2000). Living with cancer: "Good" days and "bad" days— what produces them? Can the McGill Quality of Life Questionnaire distinguish between them? *Cancer, 89*(8):1854–1865.
57. Cohen, S.R., Boston, P., Mount, B.M., & Porterfield, P. (2001). Changes in quality of life following admission to palliative care units. *Palliative Medicine 15*(5):363–371.
58. Dupuy, J. (1978, October). Self-representations of general psychological well-being of American adults. Paper presented at the American Public Health Association, Los Angeles, CA.
59. Scheier, M.F., & Carver, C.S. (1985). Optimism, coping and health: assessment and implications of generalized outcome expectancies. *Health Psychology, 4*:219–247.
60. Wyatt, G., Kurtz, M.E., Friedman, L.L., Given, B., & Given, C.W. (1996). Preliminary testing of the Long-Term Quality of Life instrument for female cancer survivors. *Journal of Nursing Measurement, 4*(2):153–170.
61. Cohen, S.R., & Mount, B.M. (1992) Quality of life in terminal illness: Defining and measuring subjective well-being in the dying. *J Palliative Care, 8*(3):40–45.
62. Padilla, G.V., Mishel, M.H., & Grant, M.M. (1992). Uncertainty, appraisal and quality of life. *Quality of Life Research 1*(3):155–165.
63. Crumbaugh, J., & Maholick, L. (1964). An experimental study in existentialism: The psychometric approach to Frankl's concept of noogenic neurosis. *Journal of Clinical Psychology, 20*:200–207.
64. Ferrans, C.E., & Powers, M.J. (1985). Quality of life index: Development and psycho-metric properties. *Advanced Nursing Science, 8*(1):15–24.
65. Flanagan, J. (1978). A research approach to improving our quality of life. *American Psychology, 33*:138–147.
66. Burkhardt, C., Woods, S., Schultz, A., & Ziebarth, D. (1989). Quality of life of adults with chronic illness: A psychometric study. *Research in Nursing and Health,* 12:347–354.
67. O'Boyle, C., McGee, H., Hickey, A., O'Malley, K., & Joyce, C. (1992). Individual quality of life in patients undergoing hip replacement. *Lancet, 339*(8801):1088–1091.
68. McGee, H., O'Boyle, C., Hickey, A., O'Malley, K., & Joyce, C. (1991). Assessing quality of life of the individual: the SEIQoI. with a healthy and a gastroenterology unit popula-tion. *Psychological Medicine, 21*(3):749–759.
69. Reed, P.G. (1991). Self-transcendence and mental health in the oldest old adults. *Nursing Research, 40*(1):5–11.
70. Antonovsky, A. (1987). *Unraveling the mystery of health: How people manage stress and stay well.* San Francisco: Jossey-Bass.
71. Paloutzian, R., & Ellison, E. (1982). Loneliness, spiritual well-being and quality of life.

In L. Peplau, & D. Periman (Eds.). *Loneliness: A sourcebook of current theory, research and therapy* (pp 224–237). New York: John Wiley & Sons.

72. Reed, P.G. (1986). Death perspectives and temporal variables in terminal illness and health of adults. *Death Studies, 10*:443–454.

73. WHO Quality of Life Group. (1993). Study protocol for the World Health Organization project to develop a quality of life assessment instrument. *Quality of Life Research, 2*(2):153–159.

74. Jacox, A.K., Bauall, B.R., & Mahrenholz, D.M. (1997). Patient satisfaction with nursing care in hospitals. *Outcomes Management for Nursing Practice, 1*(1):20–28.

75. Watson, J. (2002). *Assessing and Measuring Caring in Nursing and Health Science.* New York: Springer.

Love and Caring:
Ethics of Face and Hand*

An Invitation to Return to the Heart and Soul of Nursing and Our Deep Humanity

Jean Watson, PhD, RN, HNC, FAAN

This Appendix offers a new view of old and timeless values: the essential ethic of love, informed by contemporary European philosophies, and caring theory as well as ancient poetry and wisdom traditions. It integrates some of the philosophical views of Levinas and Logstrup with Watson's Transpersonal Caring Theory. The metaphysics, metaphors, and meanings associated with "ethics of face," the "infinity of the human soul," and "holding another's life in our hands" are tied to a deeply ethical foundation for the timeless practice of love and caring as a means to sustain not only our shared humanity but also the profession of nursing itself.

Key words: *caring, ethics of face, Levinas, Logstrup, Love, transpersonal caring theory, Watson*

Let us fall in love again
And scatter gold dust all over the world.
Let us become a new Spring
And feel the breezes drift in the heaven's scent.
Let us dress the earth in green,
And like the sap of a young tree
Let the grace from within sustain us.
Let us carve gems out of our stony hearts
And let them light our path of Love.
The glance of love is crystal dear
And we are blessed by its light.

—Rumi[1]

*Watson, J. (2002). Intentionality and caring-healing consciousness: A practice of transpersonal nursing. Reprinted with permission from *Journal of Holistic Nursing Practice,* 16(4), 12–19.

We as nurses are invited, if not required, to unite at this cross-road in nursing history, at this new century of time and confusion and questioning of nursing's survival, to reconsider what brings us together for a common purpose. Thus, this Appendix and message are not to gather up new knowledge, although they may do that, but rather they are intended to gather nursing together for a more basic common purpose: perhaps to seek what Wittgenstein called "reminders"— reminders of what we already know at some deep human, experiential level, but continually pass over in our day-to-day living.

As T.S. Eliot [2] asked in the *Waste Land and Other Poems:* "Where is the life we have lost in living? Where is the wisdom we have lost in knowledge? Where is the knowledge we have lost in information?"

It seems the task of nursing and health and healing is related to the very nature of our shared humanity. In viewing nursing at this deeper level, we realize that our jobs have been too small for the nature of our work and the needs of those whom we serve as well as too small for the evolution of our individual and collective humanity.

When working with others during times of despair, vulnerability, and unknowns, we are challenged to learn again, to reexamine our own meaning of life and death. As we do so, we engage in a more authentic process to cultivate and sustain caring healing practices for self and others. Such care and practices elicit and call upon profound wisdom and understanding, beyond knowledge, that touch and draw upon the human heart and soul.

In this reminder of basic values that transcend all circumstances and time and place, we invoke the fullest and highest spiritual, spirit-filled dimensions into our work, allowing us to engage once again in compassionate service, motivated by love, both human and cosmic. From this place we offer to ourselves, and those whom we meet on our path, our compassionate response for fulfilling our chosen life's work and calling.

Just as it is in our personal lives that during crises of illness, tragedy, loss, or impending death that we ponder spiritual questions that go beyond the physical material world, it is here in our professional life, in its conventional, dispirited, physical, technical, life-form, deathbed of sorts, that we are given new freedom, new space to reconsider a deeper level of nursing. This may be the moment to reconsider what has always been the foundation of caring and healing but must now be reconsidered again for new/old reasons. Could the professional deathbed of sorts that we face in the conventional, medical, and nursing world be an opportunity for us as professionals to consider how we may live our lives if we had "only a year to live." What and how would we approach our last year to heal and be healed with so much unfinished business accumulated during this past century? How could we offer up our heart when we may be disheartened or in fear?

As Kierkegaard[3] might say, how do we encounter our sickness unto death, in this in-between existence where spirit and matter have been torn off, split asunder, from our identity, our existence, our very being? Revisiting such foundational issues of infinity of humanity in relation to our caring may be the difference between life and death of a profession.

Having during the past few years come through a period of personal trauma and loss that was and remains deeply profound, I find that I was ironically given the gift of Spirit—the opportunity to fully experience life and spirit in raw form, in the midst of deep suffering.[4,5] But the universal lesson from Buddha is that it does not matter how long you (we) have forgotten, only how soon you (we) remember. It is as if we have to be stopped to allow our souls/our soulful purpose to catch up with us. This insight may offer a moment of enlightenment for nursing at this crossroad of its survival, which may be the gift from this passage.

Perhaps it is only when we acknowledge how much pain and suffering there is in our broken hearts and broken spirits, our broken world—within and without—that we can return to that which is timeless that can comfort, sustain, and inspire/inspirit us. It is here in this broken, wounded place that we can quiet the outer pace, bow down, and surrender to the loving presence of the universe and all its infinity.

So within this framework of caring and love, we now have a new call to bring us back to that which resides deep within us and intersects with the focus of this time and place to uncover the latent love in our caring work as well as connect us with contemporary philosophies that invite love and caring through our ethics of being–becoming. For example, the philosophy of Emmanuel Levinas[6] and his notion of the "Ethics of Face" help us connect with this ancient and contemporary truth. Likewise, I acknowledge the work of Knud Logstrup,[7] a Danish philosopher who mirrors views similar to those of Levinas but from the metaphor of "Hand," in that he reminds us that:

> holding another person's life in one's hand, endows this metaphor with a certain emotional power that we have the power to determine the direction of something in another 'person's life[;] we're to a large extent inescapably dependent upon one another[,] we are mutually and in a most immediate sense in one another's power.[7]

Perhaps it is love that underpins and connects us through our metaphors of facing and holding another in our hands, reminding us of another dimension as to how to sustain our humanity at a deeper level at this point in human history.

Josephine Hart of the *London Times* wrote a compelling article on September 19, 2001, about the events of September 11, 2001. Her article frames these issues more profoundly:

We learnt a new moral alphabet this week.

The letters which form the word love seemed empowered with more resonance, as though for all our lives we had not been spelling it correctly.

We learnt that the dying understood that they would not be forgotten and that the manner of their leaving would determine their family's ability to survive their death. We learnt that, with death crashing towards them and with no means of escape, men and women absolved their families of the edge of grief that leads to madness. They did not scream in rage "Why me?" nor babble in terror at what awaited them. They spoke a last "I love you," then turned towards their ghastly fate with unbelievable grace. They taught us another way to live and to die.[8]

With the crisis of meaning in our lives and work during this era in human history, we may paraphrase W.H. Auden to remember that, in the end, love is all that really matters. The native American Indians remind us that every day we should do an act of power and an act of beauty. By reconsidering the role and power of love, light, and beauty in our life, we bring back reminders of what is truly valuable, serving ourselves with timeless reminders that in returning to our own inner light and inner love, we offer an act of power and beauty to ourself and those whom we serve.

Perhaps the purpose of this book and my writing of it is more specifically to remind myself and others of one other basic thing: that it is our humanity that both wounds us and heals us and those whom we serve; in the end, it is only love that matters. It is in entering into and participating with the great mysteries of the sacred circle of life and death that we engage in healing.

By attending to, honoring, entering into, connecting with our deep humanity, we find the ethic and artistry of being, loving, and caring. We are not machines as we have been taught, but spirit made whole.

From Rumi in the 13th century to Levinas (1906–1995)[6] and Logstrup (1905–1981)[7] in the 20th century, we find the ancient truths of our work. We share the wisdom of these mystic poet-philosophers who captured the "Infinity and mystery of the Human soul, mirrored through the ethics of face" (Levinas' view), the fact that "we hold another's life in our hands" (Logstrup's view), and that "the glance," the mystical experience when eyes meet, is ancient Rumi's reminder of how we mirror the human soul through the eyes, the look, the glance.

In Rumi's words: "I see my beauty in you. I become a mirror that cannot close its eyes to your longing . . . . These thousands of worlds that arise from nowhere, how does your face contain them?" And "out of eternity I turn my face to you, and into eternity . . . ."[9]

How can we dare to be so bold as to bring caring and loving and infinity of souls into our lives and work and world again? Because, without returning to this ancient place of cosmic power, energy, and beauty, we are inclined toward what Levinas referred to as a "totalizing of self and other"[6]; that is, a congealing of our humanity, separating us from any connection with spirit, with infinity, with the great divine, without hope for healing and wholeness. A totalizing occurs when there is no relational engagement, no soul connection; thus, no cosmic human field to engage our shared humanity. This totalizing of self and other, this turning away from the mystery of our shared humanity and divine connection, can be an act of cruelty to self and others; an inhumane act toward human civilization itself, perpetuating more inhumane acts, violence, and destruction of human spirit in our work and world.

So rather than asking how can we dare to bring love and caring together into our lives and work, we can ask: How can we bear not to?

Levinas reminds us the Infinity of the human soul mirrors the mystery of humanity back upon itself to us, through our shared human connections, through "the face," "the glance," the facing of our own and others' shared souls as routes to this infinity and mysterious circularity of life.

To engage, to dwell in this new space of caring, living our mystery of being and dying, reveals the very situation in which we exist. This new space becomes our basic foundation for being and sustaining our humanity. This cosmic perspective, which invites spirit, mystery, and soul back into our lives and work, raises our courage to ethically engage in life and all its depths of being. Somehow, knowing that we can endure the pain, with the joy, the hurts, and humiliations, with the forgiveness and praise; the suffering with endurance, dignity, grace, and poise, is tied to our infinite capacity to love and be loved, to become love.

Emily Dickinson's "The brain is wider than the sky,/For, put them side by side,/The one the other will include/With ease, and you beside." can be paraphrased as: The heart is as wide as the sky, because it can hold pain and joy side by side.

Although we can find this deep ethic of being in Rumi, Levinas, and Logstrup and other poets and sages through the ages, we are invited now to be present to our own and others' deeply human soul conditions and connections that embrace all the vicissitudes of living and dying. As Rumi again reminds us: To die before we die—to find that delicate balance between self-discipline (dying of ego) and cosmic surrender.

Caring Moment as Radiating Field of Cosmic Love

I recently heard it said that when a nurse enters into a patient's room, a magnetic field of expectation is created. In this deeper, more expanded way of thinking about the power, beauty, and energy of love, a caring moment[10,11] becomes an energetic vibrational field of cosmic love that radiates reciprocity and mutuality that transcends time, space, and physicality, confirming and sustaining our humanity and our connection with Levinas' Infinity of the entire universe.[4,12]

The connections between caring, loving, and Infinity become the process of facing our humanity as mystery, thus mirroring humanity of self and other back on itself. Such a human-to-human act of caring within a given moment becomes a basic foundation for facing our humanity, uniting us and the cosmic energy of love, as one. In Rumi's words: "I am here, this moment, inside the beauty, the gift God has given . . . this gold and circular sign . . . . "[9]

Logstrup frames these issues and ethics of our artistry of being human, not only through the "look," the "face," the gesture, the glance, the voice, but also the Hands. He puts it this way:

> By our value/attitude to the other person we help to determine the scope and hue of his/her world; we make it larger or smaller, bright or drab, rich or dull, threatening or secure. We help to shape his world not by theories and views but by our very being and attitude toward him. Herein lies the unarticulated and one might say anonymous demand that we take care of life which trust has placed in our hands.[7]

These views remind us that one's human presence never leaves one unaffected. Expressed compassion and caring is not only the word that is spoken or the eye that sees, leading to action. The gaze itself is an expression; the word is also a gesture framed in a voice, an intonation. In the intuitive expression, what is said can be welcoming, receiving, affirming, but it also can be a careless phase, a looking away—nonfacing of another's humanity and human condition, a "totalizing of another," setting and limiting, objectifying an other rather than an honoring of the "Infinity and mystery of the human condition and humanity," a facing and connecting with the human soul and the infinity of the mystery therein. The opposite of this, a turning away from facing our humanity, can actually be an act of cruelty. So, in these deep ethical philosophical views of Levinas and Logstrup, which unite with caring theory, we acknowledge that through our very being, through our human presence toward facing self and other, we hold others in our hands, for better or for worse, either opening horizons to infinity or totalizing our own and others' humanity.

In this view of ethics and the metaphysics and metaphors of love, face, and hands, Levinas posited ethics as being beyond ontology: he placed ethics as the first principle of philosophy. It is acknowledging the ethical responsibility for the other, understood as vulnerability and proximity. In this view, love is originary. Love watches over other demands, such as justice.[13] The subject as other is an incomprehensible, infinite otherness. The human face is not a concept, it is not a figure whose message can be captured by knowledge. It is the face in its exposedness, its nudity, as an opening toward the infinite that makes the one responsible for the other.

This view is beyond philosophy; it is not an ontology, it is not a normative theory, it is a metaphysics: it explains how being-for-the-other precedes being-with-the-other. This approach critiques Heideggerian ontology by positioning ethics as preceding ontology. Within this metaphysics, we dwell in originary love, cosmic, and divine.[13]

Finally, what is traced in Levinas' Ethic of Face, in Rumi, mystic-ecstatic love and mystery, and Logstrup's holding another in one's hand is central to all professions involved in human care; it comes before and informs clinical judgments and can serve as an epistemological foundation for any clinical care.[13]

To frame these profound truths as foundational to our humanity, we can relate for new reasons to some theoretical notions of transpersonal caring:[11,14]

* Each thought and each choice we make carries spirit energy into our lives and those of others

* Our consciousness, our intentionality, our presence, makes a difference, for better or for worse

* Calmness and mindfulness in a caring moment beget calmness and mindfulness

* Caring and love beget caring and love

* Caring and compassionate acts of love beget healing for self and others

* Transpersonal caring becomes transformative, liberating us to live and practice love and caring in our ordinary lives in nonordinary ways

To enter into this new space of love, caring, hands, and heart that sustain infinity of our humanity, we can consider the following practices:

- ❄ Suspending of role and status: honoring each person, her or his talents, gifts, and contributions as essential to the whole

- ❄ Speaking and listening without judgment, working from heart-centered space, working toward shared meaning and common values

- ❄ Listening with compassion and an open heart, without interrupting: listening to another's story is a healing gift of self

- ❄ Learning to be still, to center self while welcoming silence for reflection, contemplation, and clarity

- ❄ Recognizing that a transpersonal, caring, loving practice transcends ego self and connects us human to human, spirit to spirit, where our life and work are divided no more

- ❄ Honoring the reality that we are part of each other's journey: we are all on our own journey toward healing as part of the infinity of the human condition: when we work to heal ourselves, we contribute to healing of the whole.

In conclusion, the crisis in modern medicine and health in this new millennium seems to lie in the lack of a meaningful perspective on the very nature of our humanity. It seems that somewhere along the way modern medicine has forgotten that it is grounded and sustained by and through the very nature of our being and becoming more human.

We have forgotten that we are nurtured and sustained by love, by grace, by the beauty and depth of life. We are reminded that with our wounded humanity, including our vulnerability, suffering, and joy, the light and shadows of our teeming humanity, we enter into and contribute to connecting with the infinity of the human soul, life itself, and all the vicissitudes that encompass and surround our humanity.

Addressing the role of our being and becoming more human, through the phenomenon, the metaphysics, and ethic of love and caring allows us to more fully "face our humanity." These considerations are critical to engage in healing practices for ourselves and for those whom we serve.

This process of connecting with Logstrup's and Levinas' ethic of first principle[6] of belonging-being and sustaining our humanity is the same as sustaining our dignity, our divinity—reminding us of the sacred world of the infinity of existence; thus humanity is ultimately floating in, trusting in, the spirit, energy, and grace of cosmic love.

This ethic of love and caring becomes first principle for facing and sustaining the infinity of our profession. If we follow this ethical demand, nursing has a critical role in moving humanity toward the omega point, ever closer to God and the mysterious sacred circle of living, trusting, loving, being, and dying.

I conclude with a quotation from Teilhard de Chardin:

> Love in all its subtleties is nothing more, and nothing less, than the more or less direct trace marked on the heart . . . . This is the ray of light which will help us to see more clearly.[15]

References

1. Rumi. (2001). *Hidden music* p. 117. M. Mafi, & A.M. Kolin (Trans.). Hong Kong: HarperCollins.
2. Eliot, T.S. (1934). Two choruses from "The Rock." In *The waste land and other poems,* p. 81. New York: Harcourt, Brace & World.
3. Kierkegaard, S. (1941). *Fear and trembling and the sickness unto death.* Princeton, NJ: Princeton University Press.
4. Watson, J. (1999). *Postmodern nursing and beyond.* New York: Churchill/Harcourt Brace.
5. Watson J. (2002). Illuminating the spiritual journey. Jean Watson tells her story. In P. Burkhardt, M.G. Nagai-Jacobson (Eds.). *Spirituality: Living our connectedness,* pp. 181–186. New York: Delmar.
6. Levinas, E. (1991). *Totality and infinity.* Pittsburgh: Duquesne University.
7. Logstrup, K. (1997). *The ethical demand.* Notre Dame, IN: University of Notre Dame Press.
8. Hart, J. (2001, September 19). Editorial. *The Times,* p. 9.
9. Rumi. (1999). "I see my beauty in you." In C. Barks (Trans). *The glance. Songs of soul-meeting,* p. 12. New York: Penguin Group.
10. Watson, J. (1999). Nursing human science and human care: A theory of nursing. Sudbury, MA: Jones & Bartlett.
11. Watson, J. (2002)> Intentionality and caring-healing consciousness: A practice of transpersonal nursing. *Holistic Nursing Practice, 16*(4):1–8.
12. Quinn, J. (1992). Holding sacred space: The nurse as healing environment. *Holistic Nursing Practice, 6*(4):26–35.
13. Nortvedt, P. (2001). Clinical sensitivity: The inseparability of ethical perceptiveness and clinical knowledge. *Scholarly Inquiry for Nursing Practice, 15*(3):1–19.
14. Watson, J., & Smith, M.C. (2002). Caring science and the science of unitary human beings: A trans-theoretical discourse for nursing knowledge development. *Journal of Advanced Nursing, 37*(5):452L–46L.
15. de Chardin, T. (1964). *The future of man,* p. 265. New York: Harper & Row.

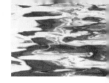

Appendix 3

Intentionality and Caring- Healing Consciousness: A Practice of Transpersonal Nursing*

Jean Watson, PhD, RN, HNC, FAAN

This Appendix explicates some theoretical and scientific dimensions of intentionality and consciousness as a framework for transpersonal nursing. New connections are made between noetic sciences and transpersonal caring theory, both of which cultivate intentionality as a form of focused consciousness as a formal field of study. What emerges is Intentional Transpersonal Caring, whereby intentionality, consciousness, and universal energy-field are posited as the foundation of a caring moment, potentiating healing for both practitioner and patient. The theoretical and scientific are translated into the practical by a series of practice guidelines that activate intentionality into a living theory of transpersonal caring-healing praxis.

Key words: *caring practice, consciousness, intentionality, noetic sciences, transpersonal caring theory*

> Intentions remind us of what is important . . . . intention
> informs our choices and our actions . . . . our intentions serve
> as blueprints, allowing us to give shape and direction to our
> efforts . . . and our lives . . . .
> —Kabat-Zinn[1]

> . . . thinking related to intentionality connects with the
> concepts of consciousness, energy . . . . if our conscious inten-
> tionality is to hold thoughts that are caring, loving, open, kind
> and receptive, in contrast to an intentionality to control,
> manipulate, and have power over, the consequences will be
> significant . . . based on the different levels of consciousness . . .
> and the energy associated with the different thoughts.
> —Jean Watson[2]

*Watson, J. (2000). Leading via caring-healing: The fourfold way toward transformative leadership. Reprinted with permission from *Nursing Administrative Quarterly*, 25(1), 1–6.

In considering the notion of intentionality, we are invited to consider/reconsider a living theory of caring in relation to our conscious living and working. To engage in this topic is to open a new horizon of meaning that embraces notions of noetic sciences as well as transpersonal dimensions of nursing. Both the noetic and the transpersonal evoke notions of consciousness and intentionality as dynamic energetic spirit manifesting transcendent aspects of being and becoming in the caring moment. This is a contemporary practice that is mindful and reflective, a practice that is graced with beauty and loving attention to our own and others' humanity. An intentional transpersonal practice emerges that cultivates a caring consciousness and the human spirit as its core, manifesting "wide awake" acts/action.

Noetic Sciences and Transpersonal Caring Theory

Noetic Perspectives

Noetic comes from the Greek *nous,* which refers to mind or direct ways of knowing.[3] Noetic sciences seek to further explorations of conventional science into aspects of reality, such as mind, consciousness, and spirit, which include intentionality; these noetic aspects of reality include but transcend physical phenomena.[3] This noetic context considers consciousness and the world of inner experience as "a promising contemporary framework within which to carry on fundamental moral inquiry."[4] One key aspect of this view is that we participate in co-creating our experiences, which arise from "thoughts as not merely a reflection on or product of reality, but also as a movement of that reality itself."[3] In other words, according to theoreticians and scientists in the field, we are urged to view consciousness (and intentionality) as critical variables, necessitating an expanded model of health and healing.[3]

In the noetic science field, consciousness and intentionality (as focused consciousness) have become a "focus of experimental research over the past 30-plus years."[3] This research to date indicates that consciousness can project itself beyond the limitations of the immediate senses.[3,4] The proliferation of interest and research in the areas of distant healing, distant intentionality, and subtle energies, as well as the influence of prayer on healing, are exemplars of renewed attention to the noetic. The noetic embraces both matter and spirit as one and invites more extended views of science than we have ever imagined. William James summed up this expanded ontology and worldview by suggesting "potential transcendence of the human spirit within the scientific study of consciousness."[3]

Transpersonal Perspective

A transpersonal perspective is related to noetic views in that both share a common interest in the theoretical concepts of intentionality and consciousness. Both perspectives embrace energy and spirit in their frameworks. Transpersonal refers to values of deep connectedness, relationship, subjective meaning, and shared humanity. Transpersonal caring theory makes intentionality, as focused caring-healing consciousness, more explicit. Thus, one's intentionality becomes activated through one's conscious focus toward aspects of reality that incorporate, but transcend, the physical as the object of attention. Transpersonal conveys a connection beyond the ego, capturing spiritual dimensions all humans share with deeper self, others, nature, and the universe.

In some ways, setting one's intentionality as a focused caring-healing consciousness of connectedness is basic to both transpersonal nursing and to the field of noetic sciences, which is the study of such focused consciousness. Thus, by integrating noetic and transpersonal perspectives, intentionality and consciousness become core concepts under a nursing framework of transpersonal caring and healing.

Definition of Intentionality

Intentionality is not the same as the word "intention," nor does it mean the same as "good intentions." Rather, the term and concept of intentionality convey a more technical, philosophical meaning referring to a consciousness and awareness that are directed toward a mental object, with purpose and efficacy toward action, expectation, belief, volition, and even the unconscious.[5-7]

When one declares intentionality toward an object or action, whatever resistance may be within tends to mobilize and dissipate, allowing manifestation of intention to be realized. Intentions do not refer to having a goal-directed outcome in mind nor a specific purpose for directing another person or situation. Rather, it is cooperating with the field, the emerging order, instead of trying to change it.[8] This line of thinking is congruent with contemporary scientific thinking, which incorporates both physical and nonphysical phenomena.[7] This integrated view of the noetic and transpersonal posits that one's intentionality and consciousness can connect with a deeper order of possibilities. One's consciousness and intentionality are posited to work within the energetic field of emerging possibilities by manifesting caring-healing consciousness within the moment.

Intentional Transpersonal Caring-Healing

When intentionality and caring consciousness are incorporated into a shared transpersonal framework for nursing practice, one begins to awaken scientifically as well as ethically. Both noetic and transpersonal views validate the importance of one's values/spiritual belief system and focused attention as a conduit to access universal life energy. This broader transpersonal field awareness of intentionality seeks to access the universal, life-spirit energy via manifesting one's deep intentional focus on a specific mental object of attention and awareness. This process invites spirit-energy to enter into one's life and work and into the caring-healing processes and outcomes.

This transpersonal, universal field view is congruent with contemporary theories of caring, as well as Rogers' science of unitary human beings.[8,9] Indeed, Smith reported that the "first constitutive meanings of the concept of caring from the Rogerian unitary perspective is *manifesting intentions*"[8] (emphasis added). In her work, she defined manifesting (caring) intentions as "creating, holding, and expressing thoughts, images, feelings, beliefs, desires, will (purpose), and actions that affirm possibilities for human betterment or well-being."[8] Other aspects of expression of (caring) intentions include: "centering on the person, preserving dignity and humanity, commitment to alleviate another's vulnerabilities, providing attention and concern, reverence for each human life, love and co-presence, approaching the other in humility, expressing compassion and courage and being with in authentic presence."[8] What emerges is an *Intentional Transpersonal Caring-Healing* practice model.

This emerging framework of Intentional Transpersonal Caring-Healing unites energy and consciousness. We realize that patterns emerge from our practices that are dynamic and energetic and that actually potentiate the caring-healing field in a given moment. It is in this space, which is created through manifesting one's caring intentions, that one witnesses safe space; sacred space[10]; authenticity; commitment; and reverence, cherishing values of love, beauty, peace, and goodness through a purposeful encounter.[8] As Smith[8] points out, during the process of manifesting intentions, one becomes more conscious, deliberate, and focused; related to expanding consciousness of unconditional love; and aware of one's integral nature, that is, one's connectedness with others, the world, and the cosmos.

This emerging interest in intentionality and consciousness also renews some of the esoteric core of religions of all worlds as well as the perennial wisdom traditions of the ages.[4] This perennial view acknowledges what Aldous Huxley noted as "a divine Reality substantial to the world of things and lives and minds . . . something similar to . . . divine

Reality."[4] The epistemology, ontology, and experience of focused consciousness and intentionality place humankind and knowledge ultimately in the realm of both the immanent and transcendent, the universal field of energy, consciousness, and spirit.[4,5]

With such an integration or synthesis of perspectives, we entertain a view whereby health and healing are acknowledged as a relational, energetic process by which individuals maintain their ability to cultivate and manifest deep values, beliefs, and meaningfulness in the midst of suffering and disease. Additional acknowledgment is given to attentiveness, presence, authenticity, personal relationships, perceptions, thoughts, and emotions as fundamental points of connection between consciousness, energy, and unitary theories and science models. This emerging focus on transpersonal caring in nursing, which is directed toward intentions and consciousness as foundational, restores the possibility of human transcendence in the face of illness, disease, suffering, vulnerability, and even death.

Such an Intentional Transpersonal Caring model now incorporates energy and universal spirit and manifests deep values of connectedness and healing. This cultivated view "now becomes primary: a source and form of life energy, life spirit, and vital energy which is connected to the energy of the universe, the universal life energy field."[5]

An Intentional Transpersonal Caring perspective becomes foundational for an ethically aware practice, which potentiates healing outcomes. An Intentional Transpersonal Caring model seeks to identify deeper sources of meaning and deeper sources of inner healing, which are defined in more spirit-filled terms than just disease elimination associated with allopathic curing.

Thus, an Intentional Transpersonal Caring field approach to healing practices requires that the practitioner pause to consider his or her own thoughts and actions in daily life. Otherwise, how is one to cultivate intentionality and an authentic caring consciousness that can manifest in one's life and work? Further, how can one consider such a daunting task?

Reconsidering Deeper-Deepest Tasks of Transpersonal Nursing[9]

When placing the notion of intentionality and caring consciousness within the context of contemporary and futuristic transpersonal nursing, we are now asked, if not required, to redefine nursing. We do that by considering the ultimate tasks of caring and healing within the intentional transpersonal vision above. Nursing for this new era can no longer be defined by a ranking order of medical procedures and bureaucratic tasks carried out as industrial employees of hospitals/institutions, but rather by inviting concepts such as intentionality, caring consciousness, energy, spirit, and transpersonal into our framework. We then hopefully can see that what we thought we were "doing" in conventional, fragmented practice models is not confined to the material world alone but belongs to something much more profound. We awaken to the fact that our jobs have been too small for the nature and needs of both those we serve and ourselves.[11]

At a deeper level, both nursing and nurses, at least within an Intentional Transpersonal Caring model, acknowledge that the model and we ourselves come face to face with humanity itself. Indeed, in this deeper, perhaps deepest view, we reveal that the tasks of humanity itself become the ultimate tasks of nursing and nurses. These ultimate tasks of nursing intersect with the following tasks of humanity (these ideas were influenced by a paper presented on spirituality by C. Lougacre in Durham, England, September 1999):

❀ Healing our relationship with self and others

❀ Finding meaning for our own life as we reawaken our profound compassion and caring for our own spiritual Journey

❀ Understanding and transforming our own and others' suffering

❀ Deepening our understanding and acceptance of all of life's cycles (the dark and the light) and preparing for our own death

In revisiting nursing's ultimate tasks within this expanding transpersonal view, nursing and nurses awaken to the ultimate concerns of humanity itself. In doing so, nurses become true instruments, embodied spirits of caring and healing. What emerges is a new vision of basic nursing practice that embraces caring consciousness, intentionality, and spirit-energy, both from within and from without. A spiritual culture unfolds of nurse-as-instrument, of "nurse as sacred healing environment,"[10] of nurse with intentional presence, engaging with grace, beauty, artistry, and loving energetic attention, not rushing, nor dismissing, nor dribbling away precious energy of healing potential. This perspective allows nursing and nurses to connect with spirit in revitalizing the spirituality in nursing.[11] This holistic view invites a living theory of caring and healing in relation to our own lives and work.[10,11] In the words of Indian writer-activist Arundhati Roy, it is "vital to de-professionalize the public debate on matters that vitally affect the lives of ordinary people."[12] Intentional Transpersonal Caring approaches affect the lives of nurses and the public alike.

Translating Theory into Action: Cultivating Our Intentionality and Caring Consciousness

As nurses working within an expanded holistic model that embraces an intentional transpersonal approach to caring and healing, we acknowledge that the tasks of nursing intersect and transform the tasks of humanity itself. We thus are challenged to reexamine our own meaning of intentionality and intentional caring practices for self as well as those we are caring for through times of suffering, despair, vulnerability, and unknowns. Cultivation of such practices elicits and calls upon profound knowledge and skills that touch and draw upon the human heart and soul. The task at hand is greater than conventional medical nursing and physical and emotional nursing care. Indeed, the task in this emerging area of Intentional Transpersonal Caring-Healing invites and evokes the fullest and highest sense of compassionate service—a service that inspires/inspirits one to grow into all of the finest aspects of living and learning a spiritual journey in one's chosen life's work and calling.

In translating the transpersonal theory into authentic practice, the mindset becomes one of creating spirit-filled sacredness and reverence around our work. We acknowledge that we are working with our own and another's life force, energy, and spirit—with human life force that has its own inner journey for living and dying. Thus, illness, pain, suffering, despair, distress, vulnerability, birthing, and dying all become an existential-spiritual human dilemma that ultimately each of us shares and must face. Consistent with timeless nursing and our Nightingale roots, we acknowledge that nursing is ultimately a spiritual practice. In acknowledging these ultimate tasks of humanity and nursing, individual nurses and nursing in general are offered an opportunity to transform practice through mindful practice as one way forward.

Cultivation of Intentionality and Caring Consciousness[11,13]

Intentionality and setting our intentions within a context of caring consciousness remind us of what is important. Our intentionalities inform our choices and actions, helping us to be sensitive and mindful about what is most important in our lives and work. Intentionality and caring consciousness converge in setting the stage for preparing ourselves for what matters and what our focus is to be and for reminding us over and over again to return to our intentions in the present: now.

Experienced practitioners of mindfulness and reflective practice remind us that it is never too late to establish this perspective in our lives and work. It means that we begin when we are ready, wherever we are, in our lives and work, in the here and now. Each of us is invited to formulate the intentions that are important to affirm and implement, intentions that are realistic and meaningful to one's own authentic value system. Not only is it never too late to begin with intentions and mindfulness, but the sages teach us that the very moment we make the conscious, intentional choice and commitment to do so becomes the perfect moment to begin.

Identify Your Own Intentions: Optional Exemplar Exercises to Point the Way

So, if and when you are ready, here are some steps and guides for cultivating and activating your intentional caring-healing practice.

* ❋ Intention One: Upon awakening each day, begin the day with a spiritual practice, even if it is being silent to receive the day and to give gratitude for life. Be open to receive the day and all the universe wishes you to receive and give in return. In this frame of mind, each morning set your intentions for the day; bring your full self, your presence-in-the-moment to your day and to your work, whatever it may be. Establish your intentions about those things you can control, letting go of those you cannot control. Be guided by caring, compassion, tenderness, gentleness, loving-kindness, and equanimity for self and others.

* ❋ Intention Two: Honor nursing as the spiritual, spirit-filled practice that it is, keeping in touch with the ancient roots of Nightingale and ancestors across time. Keep this mindfulness and intentionality alive through the use of an invocation, invoking into the space you are in the Divine source and inspiration to guide you. Invoke this higher/deeper spirit, this presence, even if you cannot see or feel it. Trust that universal Spirit resides in our lives and work.

* ❋ Intention Three: Work to cultivate discernment in your daily life and work, using an intentional awareness of the reflection and a return to the "now." It is the moment-to-moment breath that grounds and orients you to spirit, returning again and again to this intention, this mindfulness of the "eternal now" of infinite spirit. In invoking infinite spirit in the now, you invoke the notion of divine presence in all you meet, hold them in light, bless and forgive them, holding caring-healing energy in

your consciousness for both self and other. In this intentional frame, revision your place of work as a temple, a shrine, a sacred site for inner healing, taking personal "spiritual leave"[13,14] from the industrial, institutional model of sick care, doing so without bias or fear.

✿ Intention Four: Make an effort to "see" who the spirit-filled person is behind the patient or colleague. Seek to connect with others beyond the ego to the spirit-to-spirit relation in a caring moment. Offer your authentic presence, even in a brief moment, honoring the inner process that cannot be rushed, fixed, or controlled by your own or other's expectations. Trust in the ability of self and others to access the healer within.

✿ Intention Five: Use whatever presents itself in your life, including the dark and difficult times, as lessons to teach you to grow more deeply into your own humanity. Ask for help and guidance when unsure, confused, and frightened. Forgive and bless each situation, learning to surrender to that which is greater than you, and trusting spirit-filled, loving energy to flow through you for healing.

✿ Intention Six: Fold these intentions into your heart, and commit yourself to cultivating a practice of these or other heartfelt intentions as best you can, every day. In turn, you are honoring your own self and your caring consciousness-connection with these ultimate tasks of intentional transpersonal nursing and the universal healing field of possibilities. Extend your consciousness and intentions of caring and healing into your space. By bringing your authentic, intentional caring presence into your work space, you are energetically helping to repattern the environment field[10] within that moment.

✿ Intention Seven: At the end of the day, offer gratitude for all. Dedicate what you have done to the universe. Bless and forgive all that has entered into the sacred circle of your life and work. Release and dedicate the day to a deeper, higher order of the timeless cycle of the universe and the great circle of life, reminding yourself that you/we all are in the presence of that which is greater than ourselves.

✿ One last intention: Create your own intentions and your own authentic practice to cultivate caring consciousness and meaningful intentionalities. Let these practices serve as your personal guide for your own Intentional Transpersonal Caring-Healing theory in your life and work.

References

1. Kabat-Zinn, J., & Kabat-Zinn, M. (1997). *Everyday blessings* (p. 381). New York: Hyperion.
2. Watson, J. (1999). *Postmodern nursing and beyond* (p. 121). Edinburgh–New York: Churchill-Livingstone/Harcourt-Brace.
3. Schlitz, M., Taylor, E., & Lewis, N. (1998). Toward a noetic model of medicine. *Noetic Science Review, 48*:45–52.
4. Harman, W. What are noetic sciences? (1998). *Noetic Science Review, 47*:32–33.
5. Watson, J. (1999). *Postmodern nursing and beyond.* New York: Churchill Livingstone.
6. Quinn, J. (1996). The intention to heal: Perspectives of a therapeutic touch practitioner and researcher. *Advances: The Journal for Mind, Body, Health, 12*(3):26–29.
7. Schlitz, M. (1996). Intentionality and intuition and their implications: A challenge for science and medicine. *Advances: The Journal for Mind, Body, Health, 12*(2):58–66.
8. Smith, M. (1999). Caring and the science of unitary human beings. *Advanced Nursing Science, 21*(4):14–28.
9. Rogers, M.E. (1970). *A theoretical basis of nursing.* Philadelphia: FA Davis.
10. Quinn, J. (1992). Holding sacred space: The nurse as healing environment. *Holistic Nursing Practice, 6*(4):26–36.
11. Watson, J. (2001, September 13). *Reconnecting with spirit: Caring and healing our living and dying.* Presented at the Fifteenth Annual Westberg Symposium, Chicago.
12. Roy, A. (2001). *Power politics.* Cambridge, MA: South End Press.
13. Watson, J. (2001, April 30). *Creating a culture of caring.* Presented at the Creative Health Care Management Conference, Minneapolis, MN.
14. Palmer, P. (1998). *Courage to teach.* San Francisco: Jossey-Bass.

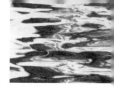

Appendix 4

Metaphysics of Virtual Caring Communities*

Jean Watson, PhD, RN, HNC, FAAN

Caring science and virtual reality both constitute a new form of human knowledge and human experience. Both have the potential to define the culture that results from their use. This Appendix explores the latest developments in caring science against some of the metaphysical aspects of virtual caring communities. Transpersonal theory and virtual concepts that transcend time, space, and physicality will be identified. The ontology of cyberspace will be uncovered against a backdrop of caring-science knowledge and practices. New territory for creating and entering virtual global caring communities will be considered as one path toward nursing and the public's future in health care.

Background of the Issues: "Space Between Life Passages"

For the past 30 years or so, the University of Colorado has hosted the annual World Affairs Conference. During this time, invited distinguished scholars, thinkers, artists, musicians, scientists, writers, political journalists, and judicial leaders come to the Boulder campus from around the globe to grapple, free-associate, and brainstorm about a plethora of contemporary and futurist issues.

During a Conference one year, I had an interesting experience. One of the invited speakers was my house guest, a retired Supreme Court justice from California. During part of the time of his stay, I had to travel to present a paper at a national conference. I explained that I was going to present a paper on "Space Life or Life Space: The Rogerian Conference on Space Nursing," held at the University of Alabama, Huntsville (which, incidentally, hosted a tribute to Martha Rogers at

Author Note This article is based on a paper presented at the International Association for Human Caring Conference, University of Stirling, Scotland, June 2001. Correspondence concerning this article should be addressed to Jean Watson, University of Colorado Health Sciences Center, School of Nursing, 4200 East Ninth Avenue, Denver, Colorado 80262. Electronic mail may be sent to Jean.Watson@uchsc.edu

*Watson, J. (2003). Love and caring: Ethics of face and hand. Reprinted with permission from *Nursing Administrative Quarterly,* 27(3), 197–202.

the joint Rogerian Conference and American Holistic Nursing Association Conference during June 2001). When he heard the topic of the conference and the title of my paper, the justice's response was, "Is that the space between life passages?"

I share this little story because of the emerging relationships between and among space life, virtual realities, cyberspace, Rogerian science, and caring science; and the wider notion, if not connection, between these concepts and the judge's innocent question, "Is that about the space between life passages?" At this moment in history, these seemingly diverse concepts and theories are converging, for perhaps new reasons.

It struck me then, and continues to impress upon me now, that perhaps his question is the right one to ask. If so, then are people (a) moving from one level of being to another; (b) evolving from a humankind to a "spacekind" form of being, as the literature suggests; or (c) evolving from *Homo sapiens* to "Homospatials," as Rogers suggested? If so, what does it all mean? What is the metaphysics of such movement between life passages and evolutionary leaps in humanity? What does this have to do with caring science? With nursing? With creating communities of caring through global initiatives?

As a starting point, when one enters into the world of global space considerations and creating virtual communities of caring, one automatically enters the metaphysical realm. By so doing, one enters into the nonphysical domain—the realm of connecting consciousness and information beyond time-space and physicality. When one introduces notions of caring and communities into the virtual realm, one is entering a reality that can and does constitute a new form of human experience—a space between life passages.

The potential impact of the shift from physical reality to virtual reality is so great that it is defining the culture that is resulting from its use, both positively and negatively. Virtual reality has already become a widely used metaphor for reality itself and for its use and practice. The virtual world has led to a change in people's relationship with technology and knowledge and, ultimately, to a change in our view of others and ourselves.

It has been suggested in some of the literature that 19th-century German philosopher and psychologist Leibniz's vision of a community of minds actually anticipated the current data web, the Internet networks, and on-line relationships (Heim, 1993). Thus, this direction has been evolving in the human consciousness as part of evolution of the species. Virtual reality itself has been traced back to hieroglyphics, to the petroglyphs, and to writing on papyrus, and it is evident in modern-day inventions such as the typewriter. As Heim points out in his book on the metaphysics of virtual reality, writing before the printing press was a form of worship. But after Gutenberg, individuals and institutions owned the written word. Thus, one revolution-evolution has led to another form of electronic, digital world and digital word, to word processing, to thought processing, and to postmodern deconstruction of text, words, and worlds.

The hypertext phenomenon breaks linear sequence, so disordered, nonlinear text replaces the straight logic of ordered thought. The reader interprets and interacts with the text, moving beyond what the author constructed, becoming part of the co-creation of the meaning of the text, beyond the original starting point of the author. This nonlinear, free-association format of hypertext, multimedia, multisensory juxtaposition of pictures and words creates a new form of expression: three-dimensional, colored, animated symbols for interaction versus an ordered, linear text that is passively read. This new order of human experiences and realities facing people in the 21st century is a quite different scenario from the mindset of the middle to late 20th century.

The paradox of virtual reality is that, on the one hand, it becomes an intelligent technique that permits active use of the body in search of knowledge and a rejoining of mind and body for a possible evolution—a new breed of evolved consciousness or intellect. On the other hand, the mind-to-mind, consciousness-to-consciousness connection in the world of cyberspace creates a disembodied human-to-human connection and, often, an intense personal intimacy with strangers and friends alike but void of an embodied physical relationship.

The status of virtual experience raises many philosophical and metaphysical questions about an evolving ontology for humankind. Some of these rhetorical but nonetheless critical questions explore the following issues: (a) the nature of relationships and the meaning behind intimacy and connection; (b) the ambiguity between fact and fiction; (c) the blurring of intimacy and ethics; (d) the disembodied knowledge, connections, and relationships; (e) the authenticity versus artificiality of experience, relationship, and expression; (f) the inversion of reality whereby the simulated reality becomes a substitute for real experience and immediacy; (g) the extent to which humans can change and still remain human; and (h) whether a new form of humanoid is emerging through a symbiosis of machine and human, whereby the human is no longer outside the computer but is a looking glass to enter into (Heim, 1993).

Thus, in this new territory one asks foundational, philosophical questions such as, "What is existence? How does one know? What is reality? Who am I? Who are you? What is space? Does space separate or connect?" These are no longer hypothetical questions, no longer remote or esoteric, but essential to consider in that they are part of the human evolution and destiny to redefine ourselves for the next leap in human experiences. As Myron Krueger says in his introduction to Metaphysics of Virtual Reality, "We have reached a point where 'what we have made, makes us'" (1993, p. ix). As humans enter into these new realities and new worlds of possibilities open to us, it brings us to a crucial point in considering these life-space passages and the relationship between space and life changes such as virtual reality and surrogate realities.

Part of what is unfolding might be thought of as a "metaphysics of being," an acknowledgement that any philosophical system expresses a truth and an apprehension of a real aspect of the reality of human life. These truths are mutually complementary. Conflict does not arise so much from the incompatibility of fundamental ideas as from the fact that different philosophical systems exaggerate one aspect of the world or human life, thus turning a partial truth into a whole or a whole into a part. Exaggerations of a philosophy serve a useful purpose. They draw attention to basic truths; once one digests the truth, then one can forget the exaggerations. Thus, one can use the truth as a source of knowledge and insight, forgetting the instrument by which it is attained. It is the metaphysical considerations of new ideas and their exaggeration to emphasize a truth that help one arrive at an insight or a new understanding.

Metaphysics pushes open the door that science and empiricism keep shut. The real role and function of metaphysics is to awaken one to an awareness of the enveloping being in which all other finite existents are grounded. It is noted that the true and primary function of philosophy and metaphysics is to awaken one to an awareness of being that transcends being; it also reminds us that no metaphysical system can possess universal validity due to the nature of metaphysics itself (Koepsell, 2000).

Definitions

Metaphysics

Just what does metaphysics mean when considering virtual reality issues and global caring communities within a caring-science context? The best discussion of metaphysics I have discovered is that of Willis Harman and his work and writing through the Institute of Noetic Sciences. For example, he points out that the word "metaphysics" has two quite different meanings (Harman, 1991, pp.5–10). The first meaning of metaphysics is a branch of philosophy that encompasses both ontology (for example, What is reality?) and epistemology (How do you know what you know?). An example might be, "I know that I am communicating with someone by sending them loving thoughts, in free space or cyberspace." The ontological question is: What and who is communicating? The epistemological questions are: Is the experience virtual or real? How do YOU know?

The second meaning of metaphysics is the study of the transcendent or supersensible, the contacting of reality that lies beyond the physical. This meaning is often associated with perennial wisdom traditions and the kind of knowledge that emerges from inward-looking, experiential, deep practice disciplines, such as meditation, yoga, or depth spiritual practices. Both meanings of metaphysics apply to virtual reality and creating virtual communities of caring at the global level. Indeed, human evolutionary leaps and cyberspace, hypertexts, and virtual, surrogate realities lead to a union of technology and metaphysics, and new considerations of the importance of caring science in nursing and health.

Transpersonal

"Transpersonal" generally refers to a human-to-human connection that goes beyond the personal, physical ego self and connects with deeper, more spiritual, transcendent, even cosmic connections in the wider universe.

Modified Ontological Assumptions

The conventional assumption of separateness—of distinct separation between observer and observed, human and nature, mind and matter, and of separation of part of a system or organism to understand how it "really works"—no longer holds in the revised view of metaphysics and the notion of transpersonal. Such separatist thinking as a foundational, ontological assumption has to be overthrown in order to comprehend, grasp, and explain virtual reality, cyberspace, and other emerging phenomena, such as distant healing and prayer research. Indeed, such thinking of separation has kept earth and heaven, human and animal, environment and nature all separate, precluding any consideration of "action at a distance," either in time or space. The interface of technology and human technology changes the basic ontological position of separation and embraces—or is required to be open to—an ontological position of unity, connectedness, and a transpersonal consciousness and technology that transcend time, space, and physicality. The result is a transpersonal, metaphysical perspective for caring science and a new foundational, metaphysical principle for considering the creation of a virtual community of caring.

Willis Harman (1991) outlined some of the aspects of self and consciousness that give new credence to the phenomenon of unity versus separation and that ultimately alter the separatist worldview or ontology to a new ontology and cosmology of unity. For example, he invited one to consider what I call the concept of transpersonal caring consciousness. The emerging unitary views, which already are upon us from the human technology symbiosis, are at odds with the outdated, conventional metaphysical assumption of separation. The implications invite new horizons of human-technology evolution, which can embrace virtual and real, nonphysical and physical caring in a new order for new meanings. They include, among other areas, the following examples as directions. First, research on creativity and intuition reveals capabilities of the hidden, intuitive mind. Also, research on out-of-body experiences and near-death experiences seems to suggest that consciousness is something other than just physiochemical processes in the brain. Third, research on multiple personality disorder, the shift from one self of consciousness to another, may be accompanied by measurable physiological changes, suggesting that personality is a holistic, nonreducible concept that can have real effects in the world *a la* Martha Rogers' theory and science of "unitary human being." Finally, lingering and growing bodies of evidence exist suggesting that the personality, in some sense, survives after physical death and may subsequently communicate back to living persons in various ways.

Considerations of Transcendence, Consciousness, or Action at a Distance

As Harman pointed out, there remain other puzzles about the metaphysics of separation that can no longer hold in a new world order of technology, cyberspace, and the virtual reality world. Elizabeth Targ's research at the University of California at San Francisco on healing at a distance and the collection of evidence Larry Dossey has compiled on prayer research become other examples of this revised ontology and metaphysical view of reality. This direction also encompasses native and ancient world traditions employing indigenous healing practices; for example, Brazilian healers' *curanderos* and other Shamanism practices around the world. In these ancient and contemporary practices, it was and is considered customary to send thoughts to others from a distance—to be in communication with a broader field of connectedness in the universe, beyond locality consciousness and even the physical, earthly plane.

Another category that upsets the separatist ontology of the metaphysics of reality is the phenomenon of "meaningful coincidences," according to one experiencing an unexpected event. Some, including Carl Jung, have referred to this phenomenon as "synchronicity," "telepathic communication," "remote or clairvoyant viewing," and connections and relationships between the act of prayer and the occurrence of the prayed-for, such as miracle healings. Although there are no "scientific" explanations of these phenomena in the conventional metaphysical frameworks of separation, there are growing explanatory models related to field phenomena, quantum physics, and mathematical devices that are all trying to link things in new ways. The result is an overturning, at some deep level, of the ontological assumption of separation and the epistemological assumption that all knowledge is based on physical-sense data. Thus, one is confronted with new phenomena, so new models with a new and old metaphysical connection of unity are beginning to be contrived to account for nonconforming events. The emerging explanatory models generally are located within a new metaphysical foundation often referred to as a "transformative unitary framework." The emerging developments in technology, the Internet, virtual realities, and cyberspace all can be thought to reside in this new framework rather than the conventional separatist ontology of reality.

When this new view of reality, virtual or otherwise, begins to embrace the phenomenon of consciousness and consciousness at a distance (for example, one can witness this emergence in the field of distance education), new rules and new metaphysical assumptions have to come into play. This shift leads one to consider virtual caring communities based upon new metaphysical, ontological assumptions of unity and transpersonal dimensions.

$E = mc^2$: Metaphysics of Transpersonal Virtual Caring Communities

"Someday, after we have mastered the winds, the waves, the tides, the gravity, we shall harness . . . the energies of love. Then for the second time in the history of the world, we will have discovered fire" (Teilhard de Chardin).

David Bodanis' latest book, $E = mc^2$, can provide some new images and concepts for these ideas of love, energy, speed, and mass, even as metaphors. For example, as he makes clear, $E = mc^2$ is translated into E/energy = mass ? celeritas/speed^2. In using the metaphor and deeper understanding of $E = mc^2$, we can posit that the intellectual exchange of ideas (consciousness) that takes place underneath, in between, or beyond the verbal, cognitive word exchange is a more fundamental energetic exchange that can be communicated beyond time and space and physicality.

To play with these ideas within a transpersonal caring framework and new metaphysics, one could suggest another version of the equation; that is, E/energy = mass (caring consciousness) × caritas/love^2 (Figure A4-1). What results is a new formula, positing transcendent speed of nonlocal caring consciousness being sent at celeritas (speed faster than light) generated by energy of caritas/love, making new connections between words, such as celeritas ? caritas. Thus, in this way one can imagine virtual caring communities as "vast energy sources" (caring-loving consciousness) hidden in solid matter itself (mass), waiting to be released into the universe. "All of mass is really part of a connected whole, which is energy ? celeritas/speed" (Bodanis, 2000, pp. 28–29).

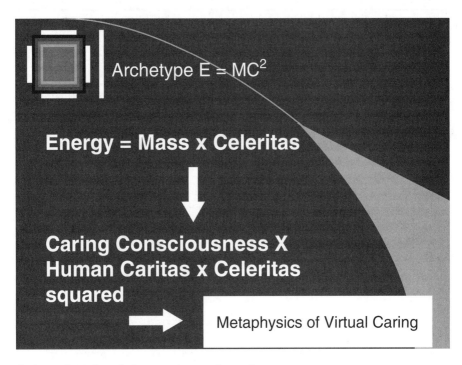

※ **Figure A4-1** Formula for metaphysics of virtual caring.

Virtual Caring and Transformative Learning

Continuing with the $E = mc^2$ thinking with respect to new learning approaches, Bache (2001) noted that in transformative (virtual caring communities) learning, words not supported by the energy of personal experiences carry much less power to influence others than words that carry energy, consciousness, and intentionality (of love and caring). He indicated that this happens partly because when people communicate in person or at a distance, they unleash a tangible but invisible power into the space around them. This power comes from experience, consciousness, and, ultimately, the energetic access that the experience has created in us. Higher energy thoughts such as love and caring carry higher frequency energy into the space, even if virtual. As Bache revealed this understanding, he suggested that words float on this power, like a canoe floating on a rushing stream.

However, in relation to caring community work, real or virtual, the power of the teacher, or faculty, or leader alone is not the only power. The more important power is the power of the group, the community, and the learning circle. Thus, the intensity and authenticity of the community's individual and collective involvement in their own learning influences the strength of the energetic stream that underpins any of the content.

In this way of thinking, people begin to envision other dimensions of space, and words and communication offer extra dimensions with infinite facets. Instead of using linear, page-by-page, line-by-line, book-by-book approaches, we now learn to connect information. We seek the "text" in the intuitive; we find the associative manner, the intentionality and consciousness behind the words. We hear the stories and engage in the relationships of patients, nurses, students, and faculty. These stories and relationships can be turned over from different angles; different twists of the same text can be deconstructed and reconstructed for deeper dimensions of insight and understanding. We in turn begin to generate new archetypes for learning. We foster creativity, critique and literacy, intuition, and leaps of imagination, prompted by energetic jumps and "aha!s" of insight and new associations. In this framework, virtual caring pedagogy can serve as a form of meditation in the sense of the Latin word *meditar,* meaning "to be in the middle of, to hover in between."

The emerging metaphysics for both real and virtual caring learning and transformation is one of wholeness, of unitary awareness of a universe that is alive, unfolding, saturated with many more hidden orders of harmony than people can imagine, opening us again to the mysterious order that is organic and integrated and that has a beautiful design that we are just beginning to grasp. Thus, within the new metaphysics of transpersonal caring and virtual caring communities, one of the key criteria is whether individual and collective learning is being pursued in a way that supports powerful, positive, and enduring life transformations in individuals and in groups, not only in those present physically but also, perhaps especially so, in those persons not physically present but virtually there.

Metaphysics of Space and Touch in Virtual Caring

In this new transpersonal metaphysics of virtual caring, space is revisioned. Space can either separate or connect people, depending upon our worldview and the metaphysical position we select. In this same way, we can rethink caring touch. Touch can occur energetically at a distance or locally in person. Touch can be experienced virtually or actually and still be effective, depending upon the energy of the consciousness behind it, namely, caring and love or indifference.

In the same line of thinking, we consider "telecaring," "telepresencing," and "teletouch," making imagination and the virtual real by not being subject to the physical world alone and its limitations. This telecaring direction, however, calls forth our creative imagination, new explanatory models, and an evolving consciousness of our own human-field possibilities. Here we realize a deep understanding of field, which encompasses both outer and inner space. For example, virtual (caring) touch embraces all the senses—auditory, voice, visual, sensory, aesthetic, imaginary, olfactory, and meaning—not just the physical body. Touch in this framework includes feelings, emotions, and perceptions, be they physical or mental or heartfelt.

However, within the model of virtual as well as physical touch, we must consider what we are intending: profane or sacred, good or harmful intentions. This heightened awareness of intentionalities becomes part of the metaphysics as well as the ethics of virtual caring communities. This framework still offers and needs to have an underlying logic, consistency, and coherence to it as part of a caring pedagogy and structure. It is here that the paradigm or framework shift is absolutely essential and must be made explicit. It, in turn, needs to be integrated, coherent, and made real in actual and virtual experiences. Because the cultural shift is rooted so deeply in our definition of reality (our metaphysics) and what is possible, a profound and comprehensive realignment of our mission and sense of self and other must be cultivated, sustained, and practiced. In doing so, we are still honoring the values and intentionalities of human preservation, human dignity, wholeness, alleviation of vulnerability, and so on. This conscious, intentional, values-based direction is intrinsic to nursing and the theory-guided practice of caring.

Finally, a new metaphysics for creating virtual communities of caring within a transformative learning paradigm is part of what is necessary for the future of nursing. What is required is to be consciously open to these potent energy sources of love and caring that are reaching into humanity from below and above. It is to consciously choose to participate, cooperate, and co-create with the creative process, making ourselves available to the rising energies of change and transformation that are fueled by a new consciousness of love and caring. It is to step voluntarily into the alchemical fire of our own energetic field resonance of celeritas and caritas.

References

Bache, C. (2001, Spring). *Transformative learning,* pp. 2–6. Noetic Sciences Institute.

Bodanis, D. (2000). *E=mc².* New York: Walker.

Harman, W. (1991). *A re-examination of the metaphysical foundation of modem science.* Sausalito, CA: Institute of Noetic Sciences.

Heim, M. (1993). *The metaphysics of virtual reality.* Oxford: Oxford University Press.

Koepsell, D.R. (2000). *The ontology of cyberspace.* Chicago: Open Court.

Krueger, M. (1993). Introduction. In M. Heim. *The metaphysics of virtual reality,* (p. ix). Oxford: Oxford Press.

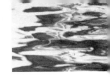

Caring Science and the Science of Unitary Human Beings*

A Transtheoretical Discourse for Nursing Knowledge Development

Jean Watson, PhD, RN, HNC, FAAN, and Marlaine C. Smith, PhD, RN

Background. Two dominant discourses in contemporary nursing theory and knowledge development have evolved over the past few decades, in part by unitary science views and caring theories. Rogers' science of unitary human beings (SUHB) represents the unitary direction in nursing. Caring theories and related caring science (CS) scholarship represent the other. These two contemporary initiatives have generated two parallel, often controversial, seemingly separate and unrelated, trees of knowledge for nursing science.

    Aim. This Appendix explores the evolution of CS and its intersection with SUHB that have emerged in contemporary nursing literature. We present a case for integration, convergence, and creative synthesis of CS with SUHB. A transtheoretical, transdisciplinary context emerges, allowing nursing to sustain its caring ethic and ontology within a unitary science.

    Methods. The authors critique and review the seminal, critical issues that have separated contemporary knowledge developments in CS and SUHB. Foundational issues of CS, and Watson's theory of transpersonal caring science (TCS) as a specific exemplar, are analyzed alongside parallel themes in SUHB. By examining hidden ethical-onto-logical and paradigmatic commonalities, transtheoretical themes and connections are explored and revealed between TCS and SUHB.

    Conclusions. Through a creative synthesis of TCS and SUHB we explicate a distinct unitary view of human with a relational caring

*Watson, J. (2002). Metaphysics of virtual caring communities. Reprinted with permission from *International Journal of Human Caring,* 6(1), 41–45.

ontology and ethic that informs nursing as well as other sciences. The result is a transtheoretical, transdisciplinary view for nursing knowledge development. Nursing's history has been to examine theoretical differences rather than commonalities. This transtheoretical position moves nursing toward theoretical integration and creative synthesis versus separation, away from the balkanization of different theories. This initiative still maintains the integrity of different theories while facilitating and inviting a new discourse for nursing science. The result: Unitary Caring Science that evokes both science and spirit.

Keywords: *Rogers' science of unitary human beings, caring science, Watson's transpersonal caring theory, unitary caring science, transtheoretical, transdisciplinary*

> While from the bounded level of our mind
> Short views we take, nor see the lengths behind;
> But more advanced, behold with strange surprise
> New distant scenes of endless science rise!
> —Alexander Pope

Introduction

The focus of this Appendix is the exploration of the evolution of CS and its relationship with SUHB. These two contemporary initiatives have generated two parallel, often controversial, seemingly separate and unrelated, trees of nursing knowledge. We offer a transtheoretical view of these two, often differing perspectives by considering commonalities. This transtheoretical view offers a new discourse for nursing science. These two directions have emerged during the past three to four decades as nursing has made great strides in its knowledge and theory building. Part of this evolution has encompassed specific caring theories as well as developments in nursing models, nursing science, and a variety of nursing theories.

Several frequently cited nursing writers represent developments of specific caring theories (for example, see earlier works of Leininger, 1978, 1990; Watson, 1979; Ray, 1981; Gaut, 1983; Gadow, 1990; Roach, 1987; Boykin & Schoenhofer, 1993; Swanson, 1999; Eriksson, 1997; Eriksson & Lindstrm, 1999). While there are various and differing perspectives on caring theory, caring itself is noted to transcend any particular model or theory and increasingly acknowledged as central to the professional discipline of nursing (Watson 1990; Newman et al., 1991; Smith, 1999).

Likewise, Rogers' SUHB has informed the work of a cadre of nursing scholars and new generations of nurses and doctoral students who adopt a unitary view of human that transcends any one nursing model or specific theory. The past tendency in nursing theory and scholarship has been to examine theoretical differences that separate rather than unite ideas, thus inhibiting creative evolution of ideas. We offer a critique and overview of CS and SUHB, which maintains the integrity of differences while also explicating shared themes that mutually inform and transform both perspectives. A transtheoretical, transdisciplinary discourse in nursing knowledge development is generated.

Background of Caring Theory and Its Evolution in Nursing Knowledge Development

Three major categories of caring knowledge development that transcend individual theories were identified by Boykin and Schoenhofer (1993) as the ontological, that is, caring as a manifestation of being in the world; anthropological, that is, the meaning of being a caring person; and ethical or obligative nature of caring. A fairly recent critique of caring research was completed by Swanson (1999). She completed a meta-analysis of 130 publications of empirical caring studies. Sherwood (1997) did a similar review by conducting a meta-analysis of qualitative studies of caring in nursing research. Their work helped to emphasize ethical aspects of caring processes and outcomes of caring in nursing and their intersection with empirical findings in the literature. For example, both meta-analyses acknowledged caring knowledge and ways of being that affect personal and professional practices, for better or for worse, for patients as well as for nurses.

These empirical findings and conceptual orientations toward caring offer some directions for substantive nursing knowledge development and locate ethical and empirical caring within the context of nursing science. Furthermore, these views of caring knowledge development help to reveal caring as a philosophical-theoretical-epistemic undertaking, not just a "nice" way of being. Rather, caring is an ethical, ontological, and epistemological project requiring ongoing exploration and expansion. As Mayeroff (1971) reminded us, we need knowledge to care.

> We sometimes speak as if caring did not require knowledge, as if caring for someone, for example, were simply a matter of good intentions or warm regard . . . . To care for someone, I must know many things . . . such knowledge is both general and specific. (Mayeroff, 1971, p. 13)
>
> Caring . . . includes explicit and implicit knowledge, knowing that and knowing how, and direct and indirect knowledge . . . . (Mayeroff, 1971, p. 15).

Critique of Caring Knowledge

In spite of the ontological, epistemological, and ethical views and diverse categories of caring knowledge, and in spite of Mayeroff's philosophical charge about needing different forms of caring knowledge (e.g., general, specific, explicit, implicit, direct, indirect), a recent publication by Paley (2001) critiqued both the pursuit of caring knowledge as well as the approaches toward development of caring knowledge in nursing. By using Foucault's archaeological view of knowledge as his lens, Paley suggests that nursing scholars' view of knowledge of caring is dated and faulty. It can be reduced to "knowledge of things said, a chain of association, constantly expanded, constantly repeated" (p. 9). His conclusion is that the effort to generate caring knowledge is for all intents and purposes unattainable: thus, caring is "an elusive concept, which is destined to remain elusive—permanently and irretrievably" (p. 9).

Paley categorized the major approaches used in the nursing literature to generate caring knowledge. For example, descriptions of caring, collection of things said about caring, knowledge of caring via association, attributes of caring and aggregation via accumulation. In his critique, he laments the fact that (1) this approach does not yield knowledge and (2) each effort leads to continued efforts to constantly retrieve caring from its elusiveness (via these varying faulty approaches), "only to return, again and again" (p. 2) to (the elusive concept) and conclude again it is elusive and needs additional study.

Paley's tautological conclusion and critique of caring knowledge is related to an earlier review by Morse et al. (1990), in which they classified diverse nursing authors' work on caring into five categories of caring: caring as human trait, caring as moral imperative, caring as affect, caring as interpersonal interaction, and caring as therapeutic intervention. Morse et al. concluded, as did Paley, that caring is left without any clarity as a concept because of its diversity.

It is important to respect the fact that both Paley and Morse et al. offer some new, provocative perspectives of information related to how caring is treated in the nursing literature. Further, these thorough, analytical critiques of caring knowledge mirror back to the profession the diversity and complexity and, yes, even more so, the elusiveness of caring. They cause nursing and caring scholars to pause and reconsider the nature of caring and knowledge.

While both these efforts to critique caring literature highlight the diversity, complexity, and scope of perspectives, both critiques ignored any examination or discussion as to the unique philosophical-ontological or paradigmatic worldviews in which the different works, or approaches to the study of caring, were located. The most serious weakness of these meta-level critiques is that they are acontextual, and aparadigmatic with respect to the moral-ontological foundation of the work. Caring looks differently depending on the ontological and ethical perspective in which the "approaches" and "categories" are located. Without specifying the ontology, one indeed cannot understand caring within it.

Foucault (1972) acknowledged that while the "group of elements formed in a regular manner by a discursive practice . . . can be called knowledge, . . . knowledge is also the space in which the subject may take up a position and speak of the objects with which he (sic) deals in discourse . . . . knowledge is also the field of coordination and subordination of statements in which concepts appear, are defined, applied and transformed . . . . lastly, knowledge is defined by the possibilities of use and appropriation offered by discourse . . . its articulation on other discourses or on other practices that are not sciences" (Foucault, 1972, p. 182, 183).

Thus, caring knowledge and its diversity and complexity can be seen in another, deeper context than Paley identifies, which is consistent with Foucault's broader view of knowledge. The above critiques did not seek to identify the underlying ethical, obligative, or ontological perspective of caring as a relational way of Being Human that engages our humanity, this being one of the most prominent core views of caring in the literature (see Smith, 1999 for a more detailed discussion of these issues). Rather, both major critiques of caring literature (Morse et al., 1990; Paley, 2001) paradoxically seemed to engage in the very exercise they critique; that is, at the meta-level, they accumulate words and total lists, categories, and approaches to study of caring. These were derived from a detached analysis of text, without an engagement of the ideas of caring or context espoused by the authors. This view of detached information is related to Lithuanian-French philosopher Levinas (1906–1995) and his critique of some of the writings of Heidegger and Husserl when he noted: "To comprehend the tool is not to look at it but to know how to handle it" (in Nortvedt, 2000, p. 6).

Foucault (1972) noted that there are dimensions (of knowledge) that are not invested in scientific discourses alone, but in a "system of . . . values . . . . an analysis that would be carried out not in the direction of the episteme, but in that of what we might call the ethical" (p. 193). Fleming's (2001) recent critique of nursing knowledge called for the notion of phronesis as a guide for critiquing nursing knowledge. He pointed out that phronesis emphasizes deliberation (reflection) and moral action, reminding us that phronesis requires that the "context of the situation be considered very carefully . . ." (p. 251) with respect to knowledge and action. Indeed, in his recent work, Nortvedt (2000) claims that "knowledge, and in particular clinical knowledge, rests on a precondition . . ." (p. 10)—the precondition being ethical sensitivity and value-laden experience.

Without addressing moral-ethical context and ontological foundations, that which results are more bits of information with a hard conclusion that has the impression of an attempt to totalize the discourse, which shuts off the debate as well as further pursuit of caring knowledge. Decontextualized bits of information, whether obtained at the specific level of analysis or at the meta-level, do not equal understanding. As Critchley (2002) emphasized in his work on Levinas, "ethics (and caring) is not a spectator sport" (p. 29). Human caring contains judgments, moral values as well as knowledge per se. There are moral, ethical insights that underpin the diverse approaches and categories, which are not acknowledged by these recent critiques of caring literature.

Thus, what is missing in these important critiques of caring in nursing literature is the fact that, first and foremost and most deeply, caring is an ethic, laden with moral values. Caring is a value-laden human condition that, according to Nortvedt (2000), is a precondition for proper clinical knowledge. Drawing upon the philosophy of Levinas (1969) we suggest the human encounter of caring exists as an "ethic of first philosophy" (Levinas, 1969) in which caring is understood (with all its categories, lists, attributes, collection of words, approaches, meta-analyses, etc.) as a value-laden relation of infinite responsibility to self and others.

We agree with Paley (2001) and Morse et al. (1990) for different reasons, that is, that engaged, ethical, value-laden caring is truly ineffable and ultimately unknowable; it is unknowable because it is an engaged moral relational human-to-human living experience that is alive in the moment, not an objective phenomenon per se. With Levinas, the infinity of other as an ethical event is the opening toward knowledge, toward epistemology, but it is not knowledge (Nortvedt 2000).

Because of the deep relational, obligative ethical nature of caring, much of the caring literature does not claim to provide us with new knowledge qua knowledge, in terms of themes or categories or even fresh discoveries. Rather, knowledge of caring is much like what "Wittgenstein called reminders, of what we already know (at some deep human experiential level) but continually pass over in our day-to-day living" (Critchley & Bernasconi, 2002, p. 10).

Levinas (1969) reminded us ethics is otherwise than knowledge (Critchley & Bernasconi, 2002, p. 15) and that ethics is not reducible to epistemology. Indeed, knowledge of caring is, like most of the important ideas in the history of humankind that seek to define and sustain our humanity, ineffable, difficult to describe, and incomprehensible.

216

However, just because concepts such as caring, suffering, love, beauty, God, and so on are "elusive," we struggle to capture their essence because of their importance. We always fall short and will continue to fall short. Nevertheless, we strive to know them through many different methods and approaches; we seek descriptions, qualities, attributes, etc. as well as how they are experienced.

Perhaps the most important conclusion with this debate is to acknowledge that caring cannot be reduced to comprehension and empirical knowledge alone that we so earnestly seek. It is perhaps because of the very reality of what Levinas framed as the "face-to-face relation." Indeed, perhaps it is because of this very elusive, deep unknowable, relational, obligatory human-to-human aspect of caring that it calls nurses paradoxically to continually pursue it. As Paley (2001) puts it: "only to return, again and again, to a concept no less ambiguous and confused, than before, the goal to all intents and purposes unattainable" (p. 2). The one-to-one human engagement in an ethical caring moment will forever remain unknowable and elusive but forever sought after, just as are beauty and truth.

Evolution of Caring Science

In spite of critiques of caring in nursing and even attempts to eliminate caring as an essential concept for nursing, we witness that over the past two to three decades the focus on caring and caring knowledge development in nursing has indeed not ceased but has even continued to accelerate. For example, the International Association of Human Caring is now into its 24th year of supporting scholarly publications and presentations. The relatively new journal *The International Journal of Human Caring* is dedicated to disseminating scholarship related to human caring. The Scandinavian *Journal of Caring Science* has been in existence since the 1980s. In 1995 the American Nurses Association revised its definition and policy statement of nursing to include caring. Major national conferences and think tanks have acknowledged caring as core in nursing theory and knowledge development (Stevenson & Tripp-Reimer, 1990).

In spite of, or because of, the still controversial unresolved discourse about caring knowledge and caring as meta-level concept for the discipline, caring has become more formalized through nursing theories and research and has been enhanced by scholarship in other related fields of study, such as ecology, education, ethics, and theology (for more information, see Mayeroff, 1971; Gilligan, 1982; van Hooft, 1995; Noddings, 1984; Watson, 2002). With this, there is a growing recognition of caring as a philosophical-ethical-epistemic field of study. As work has advanced in multiple spheres, a more formal CS framework is emerging for nursing and other related fields; thus caring scholarship has moved toward cross-disciplinary activities and intersections. For example, CS departments and academic structures for nursing have become more prominent. The field of CS has been long-standing in Scandinavian countries, e.g., Finland, Sweden, and Norway.

From a knowledge development standpoint, caring theory and knowledge are located within nursing science as well as other disciplines. Thus, caring knowledge is increasingly transdisciplinary; that is, transcending several disciplines. Caring knowledge and practices affect all health, education, and human service practitioners. Thus, CS is emerging as a distinct field of study within its own right.

Nursing's disciplinary focus on the relationship of caring to health and healing differentiates it from other disciplines that relate caring to the unique concerns of their domain. However, because of recent transdisciplinary developments in caring scholarship, it is helpful to identify some major foundational assumptions that seem to inform CS and scholarship.

A working set of assumptions for CS include the following:

❊ Developing knowledge of caring cannot be assumed; it is a philosophical-ethical-epistemic endeavor that requires ongoing explication and development of theory, philosophy, and ethics, along with diverse methods of caring inquiry that inform caring-healing practices.

❊ Caring science is grounded in a relational ontology of unity within the universe (in contrast to a separatist ontology that guides conventional science models); this relational ontology of caring establishes the ethical-moral relational foundation for CS (and for nursing) and informs the epistemology, methodology, pedagogy, and praxis of caring in nursing and related fields.

❊ Caring science embraces epistemological pluralism, seeking the underdeveloped intersection between arts and humanities and clinical sciences, which accommodates diverse ways of knowing, being-becoming, evolving; it encompasses ethical, intuitive, personal, empirical, aesthetic, and even spiritual/metaphysical ways of knowing and being.

❊ Caring science inquiry encompasses methodological pluralism whereby the method flows from the phenomenon of concern, not the other way around; the diverse forms of caring inquiry seek to unify ontological, philosophical, ethical, and theoretical views while incorporating empirics and technology.

A Working Definition of Caring Science

Caring science is an evolving philosophical-ethical-epistemic field of study that is grounded in the discipline of nursing and informed by related fields. Caring is considered by many as one central feature within the metaparadigm of nursing knowledge and practices. The development of CS is informed by an ethical moral stance with a relation of infinite responsibility to other human beings (Levinas 1969); this view encompasses a humanitarian, human science orientation to human caring processes, phenomena, and experiences. It is located within a worldview that is nondualistic, relational, and unified, wherein there is connectedness of all. This worldview is sometimes referred to as a unitary transformative consciousness paradigm (Newman et al., 1991; Watson, 1999), nonlocal consciousness (Dossey, 1991), and Era III medicine/nursing (Dossey, 1991, 1993; Watson, 1999).

Caring science thus intersects with the arts and humanities and related fields of study and practices, including, for example, ecology, peace studies, philosophy-ethics, women/feminist studies, theology, education, and mind-body-spirit medicine and the growing field of complementary medicine, health, and healing.

Reconciling Caring Dissonance: Within the SUHB and Nursing Metaparadigm

While CS, including caring theories in nursing, has been emerging over these past decades, Rogerian science has escalated as preeminent, revolutionizing nursing as well as related disciplines. There has been, however, little integration of the common foundational elements of CS and SUHB.

Indeed, as already highlighted through the critiques of Morse et al. (1990) and Paley (2001), the inclusion of caring as a central and defining concept within the discipline of nursing continues to be contentious (Smith, 1999). Rogers had serious concerns about caring being named within nursing's metaparadigm or as part of the essence of nursing. She was concerned that it would not advance the discipline of nursing nor generate substantive knowledge for practice.

Rogers' worldview offered and continues to offer a new vision and conceptual system for generating and addressing phenomena related to unitary life processes. Thus, Rogers viewed caring as an important stance in the practice of any human service field but not as a substantive area of knowledge development for nursing (Smith, 1999).

What is more significant within the area of theory and knowledge development is the fact that CS and SUHB have coexisted over these past few decades almost as two separate trees of knowledge. Both areas were pursuing their individual interests without exploring the common philosophical-ontological foundation and scientific assumptions that they may share. These common foundations may strengthen the advancement of nursing knowledge for this new century. For example, both the Society of Rogerian Scholars and the International Association of Human Caring hold scientific sessions. The papers presented have overlapping themes and yet there is little to no connection or communication between the two scientific groups.

This dissonance between CS and SUHB, including the ambivalence about caring and its location with the disciplinary matrix of nursing, is still a tense undercurrent in nursing knowledge development circles. However, there are some noted exceptions.

Newman et al. (1991) offered a significant contribution to the evolution of including caring within the disciplinary matrix by acknowledging in their critique of the existing metaparadigm that caring and health are linked within the theoretical literature of nursing. They then posed a manifesto of sorts with their well-known statement that sought to integrate caring into the metaparadigm: "Nursing is the study of caring in the human health experience" (Newman et al., 1991, p. 3).

Further, they acknowledged the use of different paradigms for knowledge claims and explication of (caring) knowledge. The three well-known paradigms they named are:

❋ Particulate-deterministic: isolated phenomena, reducible entities with definable measurable properties

❋ Interactive-integrative: extension of particulate-deterministic plus context, experience, and subjective data

❋ Unitary-transformative: representing a significant paradigm shift whereby phenomena are viewed as unitary and self-organizing, embedded in a larger self-organizing field that is whole and unified.

Another major work that attempted to explore new relationships between caring knowledge and its paradigm location is Smith's seminal work in 1999. She tried to break the exclusivity of these two separate trees of knowledge development within nursing, i.e., CS and SUHB.

Smith (1999) "critiqued the critique" of caring in nursing. In contrast to Paley (2001) and Morse et al. (1990), Smith located consistent ontological perspectives from extant caring theory within SUHB. By working at the ontological-ethical level she was able to clarify how caring resides within SUHB; she explicated points of congruence between existing literature on caring and shared meanings in SUHB.

Smith identified five constitutive meanings of caring from a wide range of caring theories. Each of these meanings was conceptually located within the SUHB system: (1) caring is a way of manifesting intentions; (2) caring is a way of appreciating pattern; (3) caring is a way of attuning to dynamic flow; (4) caring is a way of experiencing the infinite; (5) caring is a way of inviting creative emergence.

Smith (1999), Watson and Smith (2000), and earlier work of Newman et al. (1991) attempted to extend the discourse about caring at the metaparadigm level. These works reflect the commonalities of a caring ontology that apply to a range of caring theories. Further, both locate particular scholarship on caring and SUHB within the unitary-transformative framework, i.e., "patterning, dynamic flow, manifesting intentions, and experiencing the infinite"; these features go beyond conventional particulate or interactive models for explaining phenomena, reflecting a worldview that resides within the unitary-transformative paradigm.

This next section seeks to extend these intersecting connections between CS and SUHB within the unitary-transformative paradigm. An overview of Rogers' SUHB will be followed by a summary of one specific theory of caring: Watson's transpersonal caring theory. The transpersonal caring theory will be used as an exemplar for the CS model to reflect the intersections with Rogers' SUHB.

By expanding the discourse on nursing knowledge development, a new evolution for nursing—caring knowledge and transtheoretical theory development—unfolds. Further, by exploring the convergence of ideas within the two systems, there is advancement of knowledge that transcends nursing and contributes to a transdisciplinary future for nursing in the wider arena of human health science.

Overview of Rogerian SUHB

Parallel with and prior to the evolution of caring theories in nursing, and the emergence of CS as a field of study was the renowned work of Rogers (1970). Her views of nursing science and the concept of SUHB (Rogers, 1970, 1992, 1994) were posed as the disciplinary focus for nursing.

A review of basic principles of SUHB is offered as a contextual backdrop for examining how the two specific systems can converge and extend each other for new possibilities. Rogerian science, from its inception, was located within the now emerging unitary consciousness worldview, labeled by Newman et al. (1991) as unitary-transformative: that is, phenomena are viewed as a unitary, self-organizing field, embedded in larger self-organizing field, recognized by pattern interaction within the whole.

Tenets of Rogerian SUHB and the unitary-transformative paradigm (Barret, 1990; Rogers, 1992) are shown in Table A5-1. Rogers' work initiated a new paradigm for nursing science. For example, her theoretical basis for nursing makes explicit the connectedness of all, a unitary, irreducible mutual human-environmental field process. Further, her introduction of energy field as the fundamental unit of the living and nonliving, making "energy field" an explicit unifying concept was revolutionary in its time.

The evolution within science itself corresponds with the ontology worldview articulated by Rogers (1970). This revolutionary ontology propagates changes in epistemology, methodology, and practice that are consonant with it. To further explore the specific ontological connections between SUHB and CS, it is helpful to highlight the internal features of CS vis-à-vis a specific caring theory.

Table A5-1

Tenets of Rogerian Science of Unitary Human Beings

Energy field	The fundamental unit of the living and the nonliving. Field is a unifying concept. Energy signifies the dynamic nature of the field; a field is in continuous motion and is infinite.
Environment (environmental field)	An irreducible, indivisible, pandimensional energy field identified by pattern and integral with the human field.
Pandimensionality	A nonlinear domain without spatial or temporal attributes.
Pattern	The distinguishing characteristic of an energy field perceived as a single wave.
Principle of Resonancy	Continuous change from lower to higher frequency wave patterns in human and environmental fields.
Principle of integrality	Continuous mutual human-environmental field processes.
Unitary human beings (human field)	An irreducible, indivisible, pandimensional energy field identified by pattern and manifesting characteristics specific to the whole and which cannot be predicted from knowledge of the parts.

Caring Science and SUHB: Transpersonal Caring Theory as Exemplar

Watson's theory of transpersonal caring (Watson, 1979, 1985, 1988, 1995, 1999) is one extant caring theory among others that has emerged as a guide to practice and education for nursing and related fields. In addition, transpersonal caring serves as a disciplinary framework to guide knowledge development related to both nursing and the emerging transdisciplinary field of CS. Transpersonal caring theory is located within a CS framework. The next section provides an overview of some of the basic ingredients of transpersonal caring theory. For heuristic purposes it will be referred to as transpersonal caring science (TCS) to demonstrate parallel and intersecting connections with SUHB. Central tenets of TCS are:

❀ The transpersonal caring field resides within a unitary field of consciousness and energy that transcends time, space, and physicality (unity of mind-body-spirit nature universe).

❀ A transpersonal caring relationship connotes a spirit-to-spirit unitary connection within a caring moment, honoring embodied spirit of both nurse and patient, within the unitary field of consciousness.

❀ A transpersonal caring moment transcends the ego level of both nurse and patient, creating a caring field with new possibilities for how to be in the moment ["the process goes beyond itself, and becomes part of the life history of each person, as well as part of the larger, deeper complex pattern of life" (Watson, 1985, p. 59)].

❀ A nurse's authentic intentionality and consciousness of caring has a higher frequency of energy than noncaring consciousness, opening up connections to the universal field of consciousness and greater access to one's inner healer.

❀ Transpersonal caring is communicated via the nurse's energetic patterns of consciousness, intentionality, and authentic presence in a caring relationship.

❀ Caring-healing modalities are often noninvasive, nonintrusive, natural-human, energetic, environmental field modalities.

❀ Transpersonal caring promotes self-knowledge, self-control, and self-healing patterns and possibilities.

❀ Advanced transpersonal caring modalities draw upon multiple ways of knowing and being; they encompass ethical and relational caring along with those intentional consciousness modalities that are energetic in nature, e.g., form, color, light, sound, touch, visual, olfactory, etc., that potentiate wholeness, healing, comfort, and well-being.

Transpersonal Caring Science and SUHB

Drawing upon the above assumptions from TCS, it is now possible to extend more explicitly Smith's (1999) previous integration of caring and SUHB. For example, the following unifying statements amplify the integration of TCS and SUHB:

❊ The intention of transpersonal caring expands in open, resonating, concentric circles from self to other to Planet Earth to universe. It includes caring consciousness and participating knowingly in human-environment energy field patterning

❊ The nurse's authentic presence, consciousness, and intention in a caring moment manifests caring field patterning

❊ The nurse's presence and caring consciousness potentiate change in the field by co-creating human-environment patterning from lower frequencies to higher frequencies (i.e., caring consciousness carries higher energy frequencies than noncaring consciousness)

❊ Transpersonal caring resides within a field of caring consciousness and energy that transcends time, space, and physicality and is one with the universal field of consciousness (spirit)— the infinite.

Through this process, we find shared notions of the concepts in both the SUHB and TCS in Table A5-2.

To see a World in a Grain of Sand
And a Heaven in a Wild Flower,
Hold infinity in the palm of your hand and Eternity in an hour.
—William Blake

SUHB and TCS: Transtheoretical Integration and Extensions of Shared Commonalities

In considering transpersonal caring as an exemplar of CS that intersects with some foundational aspects of SUHB, we find harmony in diversity that can advance the transtheoretical discourse in theory and knowledge development in nursing science. In exploring relationships

Table A5-2

Shared Notions of the Concepts in SUHB and TCS

ROGERS SUHB	WATSON'S TCS
Pandimensionality	Transpersonal: transcends time, space, physicality, is grounded in the "eternal now" of the caring moment
Infinity	Universal field of consciousness: connects with infinity
Resonancy	Consciousness is energy: caring consciousness manifests high frequency energy waves
Body: manifestation of energy field	Postmodern body = light, energy, consciousness (body resides in universal field of consciousness; see Watson, 1999)
Integrability (mutual human-environment field process)	Mutuality of caring relationship within caring field
SUHB: Healing modalities: noninvasive, meditative modalities, energy-guided processes, therapeutic touch, healing environments: light, color, harmony, intentional mutual patterning of human-environmental field; pattern manifestations appraisal and repatterning	TCS: Caring-healing modalities: ethical relational, and energetic through caring consciousness, intentionality, presence, authenticity; noninvasive, nonintrusive, natural-environmental healing modalities; those modalities that help to connect with universal field to access inner healer; intentional conscious use of form, color, light, energy, sound, touch, visual, consciousness, etc.

between the parallel nursing theoretical structures, we find philosophical and theoretical convergence. Some of the more specific commonalities between SUHB and TCS are as follows:

❋ Both TCS and SUHB reside within a unitary-transformative paradigm, honoring the universal oneness and connectedness of all.

❄ Both TCS and SUHB share unitary perspectives related to mutuality of human (caring) processes, whereby a caring moment potentiates the emergence of a new human-environmental energy field pattern.

❄ Both TCS and SUHB are commingled and extended by integrating principles of energy and resonancy (from SUHB) with caring consciousness (from TCS). For example, we extend SUHB by asserting from TCS that the *caring consciousness of the nurse is a higher human-environmental field wave pattern than that of noncaring or ordinary consciousness. We extend TCS by integrating principles of resonancy into caring consciousness and caring field. Further, we make significant connections between SUHB and TCS by attending to the human-environmental field pattern co-created with the one-caring and the one-cared-for. (*Note: Rogers did not incorporate consciousness into her system; the relationship between consciousness and energy is emerging within transpersonal caring theory as well as mind-body science.)

❄ By relating transpersonal (caring) consciousness from TCS with pandimensionality from SUHB, we better understand that caring consciousness transcends time, space, and physicality and is open and continuous with the evolving unitary consciousness of the universe.

❄ By acknowledging caring as the ethical and moral foundation from TCS and relating that to SUHB, we make explicit the imperative of an ontological-philosophical view for nursing, committed to knowledgeable, compassionate human service.

❄ Drawing from both SUHB and TCS, we make explicit an expanded view of what it means to be human, thereby acknowledging the unitary, transpersonal, evolving nature of humankind, both immanent and transcendent and continuous with the evolving universe.

❄ When the energy field of SUHB and its continuous, infinite motion is integrated with TCS, we see the connection with the mystery, the infinite, the universal field of cosmic consciousness energy, of living and nonliving.

❄ By integrating consciousness and energy from the two systems, we evolve a unitary caring science that affirms a deep relational ethic and spirit that transcend all duality, thus invoking the infinite, which in turn invites the sacred to return to our profession and our practices.

❁ When nursing evolves to a point whereby it can embrace a model of knowledge development that includes both science and spirit and incorporates both caring and unitary perspectives, we enter into a new level of deep knowing about the nature of reality. This turn makes explicit an expanding unitary, energetic worldview with a relational human caring ontology. As we evolve as a profession and discipline to this new level, we are invited to consider new ways of knowing, being-becoming, and doing as unitary caring human beings in continuous relation with an evolving universe.

❁ It is here in this new turn that caring and nursing knowledge development is transformed from fragmented bits of information into a unified framework for deep wisdom; here is where we more fully can experience and accommodate the empirical with the invisible; the subtle essence of the whole universe within each caring moment. It is here in these deeper dimensions that we are invited to explore the mystical with the empirical, the transcendent with the immanent, the embodied spirit of energy and consciousness and how they potentiate and mediate health and healing for self and others. If nursing continues to mature toward this deep nondualistic knowing, we shift from material particulate medicine/nursing to nonphysical phenomena and healing processes that require new visioning, deep knowing, imagination, and creative transtheoretical emergence for an open universe of possibilities.

Policy and Practice Implications

The policy and practice implications of this discourse result in further movement toward transtheoretical and transdisciplinary approaches and alliances in both scholarship and practice. By examining consistent ideas across theories that are located within the same paradigmatic perspective, nursing moves away from fixed categories that set the debate and balkanize theoretical developments. By pursuing unities rather than theoretical differences, nursing avoids locking theories into isolated "silos" where there can be little dynamic flow. The movement toward transtheoretical integration and creative synthesis still maintains the integrity of each theory while enabling nurses to join together on policy and practice issues that are important to multiple groups (e.g., International Association of Human Caring; Society of Rogerian Scholars; International Holistic Nursing Groups and Organizations; International Reflective Practice Conference Groups, etc.). Furthermore, such efforts can unite nurses from different specialties, and even subspecialty groups to participate in transtheoretical discourse and study by generating research/scholarship teams that cut across conventional units and systems. New theory-guided practice models may emerge that integrate and synthesize unitary caring from two theoretical approaches that are internally consistent, thereby facilitating implementation and evaluation of advanced practice professional nursing qua nursing models.

Moreover, and most importantly, the transtheoretical directions of CS and SUHB are congruent with the deep relational ethical caring covenant that nursing has held with its public across time around the world. By pursuing transtheoretical unitary caring scholarship and practice, nursing is helping to sustain and live out its highest commitment to humankind and society.

Conclusion

Creative synthesis of TCS and SUHB can facilitate new directions for transtheoretical knowledge development. The integration and extension of two previously disparate trees of nursing knowledge development invite ethical-ontological and epistemological scholarship for further inquiry. By integrating nursing's unique TCS ontology with SUHB, we point toward a new transtheoretical discourse for nursing knowledge that is both discipline-specific and transdisciplinary in nature. In doing so, nursing's unique knowledge of transpersonal caring for unitary human beings can inform and extend other health and human service fields. Further, transtheoretical scholarship can generate advanced theory-guided practice models that creatively unite ideas rather than lock theories into fixed boxes, inhibiting their application and evolution.

Finally, as the search for transtheoretical meaning continues, a Unitary Caring Science emerges. Together, TCS and SUHB knowledge can advance contributions to humankind. Ultimately, while never fully comprehending the "elusive" infinity of relational human caring, these continuing pursuits help to sustain nursing's relational caring ethic of infinite responsibility to other and humanity itself. One of Martha Rogers' hopes for the open-ended nature of all of science was that knowledge would continue to evolve to benefit the care of people in an ever-changing world (Rogers, 1992).

References

Barret, E.A.M. (Ed.). (1990). *Visions of Rogers' science-based nursing.* New York: National League for Nursing.

Boykin, A., & Schoenhofer, S. (1993). *Nursing as caring.* New York: National League for Nursing.

Critchley, S. (2002) Introduction. In S. Critchley, & R. Bernasconi (Eds.). *The Cambridge companion to Levinas*. Cambridge, MA: Cambridge University Press, in press.

Dossey, L. (1991). *Meaning and medicine*. New York: Bantam.

Dossey, L. (1993). *Healing words*. San Francisco: Harper.

Eriksson, K. (1997). Caring, spirituality and suffering. In S. Roach (Ed.), *Caring from the Heart: The convergence of caring and spirituality*, pp. 68–84. New York: Paulist Press.

Eriksson, K., & Lindstrm, U. (1999). *A theory of science for caring science*. Hoitotiede 11, 358-364.

Fleming, D. (2001). Using phronesis instead of "research-based practice" as the guiding light for nursing practice. *Nursing Philosophy 2*, 251–258.

Foucault, M. (1972). *The archeology of knowledge* (A.M. Sheridan Smith, Trans.). New York: Pantheon Books.

Gadow, S. (1993). Covenant without cure: letting go and holding on in chronic illness. In J. Watson, & M.A. Ray (Eds.), *the ethics of care and the ethics of cure: Synthesis in chronicity*, pp. 5–14. New York: National League for Nursing.

Gaut, D.A. (1983). Development of a theoretically adequate description of caring. *Western Journal of Nursing Research 5*, 313–324.

Gilligan, C. (1982). *In a different voice*. Cambridge, MA: Harvard University.

van Hooft, S. (1995). *Caring: An essay in the philosophy of ethics*. Boulder, CO: University Press of Colorado.

Leininger, M. (1978). *Tran-cultural nursing*. New York: John Wiley and Sons.

Leininger, M. (1990). Historical and epistemologic dimensions of care and caring with future directions. In J.S. Stevenson, & R. Tripp-Reimer (Eds.), *Knowledge about care and caring: State of the art and future developments*, pp. 19–31. Kansas City, MO: American Academy of Nursing.

Levinas, E. (1969). *Totality and infinity*. A. Lingis. (Trans.). Pittsburgh, PA: Duquesne University.

Mayeroff, M. (1971). *On caring*. New York: Harper & Row.

Morse, J.M., Solberg, S.M., Neander, W.L., Bottorff, J.L., &Johnson, J.L. (1990). *Concepts of caring and caring as concept. Advances in Nursing Science 13*, 1–14.

Newman, M.A., Sime, A.M., & Corcoran-Perry, S.A. (1991). *The focus of the discipline of nursing. Advances in Nursing Science 14*, 1-6.

Noddings, N. (1984). *Caring*. Berkeley, CA: University of California Press.

Nortvedt, P. (2000). Clinical sensitivity: The inseparability of ethical perceptiveness and clinical knowledge. *Scholarly Inquiry for Nursing Practice 14*, 1–19.

Paley, J. (2001), An archeology of caring knowledge. *Journal of Advanced Nursing 36*, 188–198.

Ray, M.A. (1981). A philosophical analysis of caring within nursing. In M.M. Leininger (Ed.), *Caring: An essential human need*, pp 25-36. Thorofare, NJ: Slack,Inc..

Roach, S. (1987). *The human act of caring*. Ottawa, Canada: The Canadian Hospital Association.

Rogers, M.E. (1970). *An Introduction to the theoretical basis of nursing*. Philadelphia: FA Davis.

Rogers, M.E. (1992). Nursing science and the space age. *Nursing Science Quarterly 5*, 27–34.

Rogers, M.E. (1994). The science of unitary human beings: Current perspectives. *Nursing Science Quarterly 2*, 33–35.

Sherwood, G.D. (1997). Metasynthesis of qualitative analysis of caring. *Advances in Nursing Science 3*, 32-42.

Smith, M. (1999). *Caring and science of UHB. Advances in Nursing Science 21*, 14–28.

Stevenson, J.S., & Tripp-Reimer, T. (Eds.), (1990). Knowledge about care and caring. In

Proceedings of a Wingspread Conference, 1–3 February 1989. Kansas City, MO: American Academy of Nursing.

Swanson, K. (1999). What is known about caring in nursing science? In A.S. Hinshaw, S. Fleetham, & J. Shaver (Eds.), *Handbook of clinical nursing research,* pp. 31-60. Thousand Oaks, CA: Sage.

Watson, J. (1979). *Nursing: The philosophy and science of caring.* Boston: Little Brown.

Watson, J. (1985). *Human science and human care.* Norwalk, CT: Appleton-Century.

Watson, J. (1988). New dimensions of human caring theory. *Nursing Science Quarterly 1,* 175–181.

Watson, J. (1990). Caring knowledge and informed moral passion. *Advances in Nursing Science 13,* 15–24.

Watson, J. (1995). Nursing's caring-healing paradigm as exemplar for alternative medicine. *Alternative Therapies 1,* 64–69.

Watson, J. (1999). *Postmodern nursing and beyond.* Edinburgh, Scotland/New York: Churchill-Livingstone/Harcourt Brace.

Watson, J. (2002). Caring and nursing science: Contemporary discourse. In J. Watson (ed.), *Assessing and measuring caring in nursing and health,* pp 11–19. New York: Springer.

Watson, J. & Smith, M. (2000). *Revisioning caring science and the science of unitary human beings.* Paper presented at Boston Knowledge Development Conference, Boston, MA.

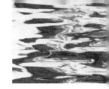

Appendix 6

Leading Via Caring-Healing: The Fourfold Way Toward Transformative Leadership*

Jean Watson, PhD, RN, HNC, FAAN

This Appendix explores an inner path of transformative leadership, guided by caring and healing. This fourfold path for visionaries, healers, teachers, and leaders converges with caring-healing practices rooted in nursing's history and its most contemporary theories. Together, they serve to remind us about the purpose of our work and how our life can speak through compassionate administrative service. This fourfold path of leading, embedded in the hidden meaning of the word *vocation* (Latin for "voice," as in giving voice to inner calling of caring-healing), may be the primary source of nursing's survival in this 21st century.

Key words: *caring-healing, Via Creativa, Via Negativa, Via Positiva, Via Transformativa*

In this waning hour of an outmoded era of nursing administration and health delivery that seeks sick and well care reform—an outdated era that applies economic indicators of care that view control, management, and health maintenance as cost containment; that acknowledges uncertainty, chaos, and complexity as a threatening norm; that is confused, if not hostile, to models of alternative-complementary medicine; that has distorted authentic caring practices—how is it that nursing administrators can survive? Especially, how can nursing administrators and leaders survive with their own vocational voice and form of authentic leadership that sustain systems of caring and healing? How can they remain intact with their own values? How can they sustain coherence and integrity for self, system, and society in a postmodern world that is turning upside down and inside out, seeking a new order in human health?

One way, one path, one road is the road less taken. The road I am referring to actually has four directions, four paths toward caring and healing, for self and system; this so-called fourfold way is inherent in any true transformative, visionary leadership.

*Watson, J., & Smith, M. (2002). Caring science and the science of unitary human beings: A trans-theoretical discourse. Reprinted with permission from *Journal of Advanced Nursing,* 37(5), 452-461.

Matthew Fox describes this fourfold path as the four *Via*.[1] It is a personal-professional journey through the four sacred directions of life itself, ultimately leading to a new horizon, a new clearing, and a new vision of hope. This fourfold way—the path, the Via—can inform nursing administrators as they seek another way through the chaos and confusion during this critical transition and provide a turning point in health and human history.

Via Negativa

The *Via Negativa* is the path of acknowledging the shadow side of our lives and work. It requires going into the dark, shadowy side of our issues, realizing that we have been in an institutional desert during this modern era and have depleted ourselves and our systems of the human spirit that sustains and heals. From "daring the dark," as Fox says, we can put new light on our obstacles and difficulties. This path of entering and daring the dark, dealing with and naming the *negativa,* also allows us to enter and dwell in the space in which germination and patience reside, the space from which new life comes from the dark time of dormancy.

Nursing's dormant, value-based vision of caring and healing and wholeness is emerging from the dark side of history to help to reestablish light and balance in systems and society that are out of balance. As nursing leaders rethink nursing's place and purpose, nursing is about to emerge from the dark and reenter the health care arena at this turning point in history. As it does, we see that new life, new germination, and new light are being brought into those spaces and places where there has been institutional darkness. Nursing's value-guided vision of care-caring for the human condition, for the embodied spirit seeking wholeness and healing, must gain voice as part of nursing leaders' true vocation.

From this *Via Negativa* nursing leaders can acknowledge that nursing and its phenomena of caring and the human health-illness healing experience embrace the dark and light as the paradox of existence for both self and system. By the *Via Negativa* nursing and nursing leaders draw upon the ancient voices from the past, from our ancestors, the mythological ancient ones who are the guardians of Mother Earth. From this rich heritage nursing leaders call upon and bring forth healing energy from the four sacred directions—North, South, East, and West. These symbolize the primary elements of the universe, earth, air, fire, and water, which are essential for the survival of humanity and planet Earth alike.

Angeles Arrien suggests that this *Via Negativa* is the way of the (spiritual) warrior.[2] Through this path, this *Via,* we are called "to show up and choose to be present" to our purpose, authentically available and mindful of that which calls us toward compassionate service. This *Via* honors the shadow aspects, the wounded aspect of our self and our systems. This *Via* gives new voice and meaning to nursing's call to care in systems and settings in which care is perverted into slogans and platitudes and transmuted into economic jargon. Underneath there is a deep institutional and human wound needing to be named in order for deep healing to occur at this time of crisis of noncaring in schools, systems, and society alike. By following the *Via Negativa* we are led to the next path, the *Via Positiva*.

Vial Positiva

By following this path nursing leaders can pause with gratitude for the special blessings, the privileged space and place we hold in the lives of humans and systems alike. It is by this path of bringing forth the light of positive, loving, caring energy into our work and world, wherever we may be, that we are replenished, and in turn we are more able to replenish others. As Fox said, by *Via Positiva* we can remind ourselves to "fall in love at least three times a day." This can occur whether it is falling in love with the new spring leaf on the budding tree, the snow flake on the eyelash, the miracle of the breath of life itself, or the look in the face of a friend, colleague, or patient that conveys the love and depth of human spirit, revealed whole to us in a given moment.

Once we open to the *Via Positiva* we can find caring moments of joy and beauty, grace and gratitude, throughout all our day, every day. *Via Positiva* is an awakened consciousness that opens our hearts to carry the joyous-sad heart paradoxically side by side, honoring the grace of both dark-light as the yin-yang of the human condition.

Through nursing leaders' ability to dwell in the grace and gratitude of the gifts of caring and healing they offer human contact, human-to-human connection, creating healing environments, becoming ontological artists and architects,[3] creating spaces and a professional culture whereby caring-healing practices flourish. Through this path of *Via Positiva* nursing leaders and administrators are nourished by the reciprocal processes of caring-healing. Thus, new energy, new light, new positive creations, and original solutions are more able to emerge from walking this *Via*.

Arrien's fourfold path corresponds to *Via Positiva* through what she acknowledges as the Way of the Healer—one who pays attention to what has heart and meaning. One takes this path from the inside out, finding one's own inner voice and unique gifts. That path in turn translates this inner voice into informed, compassionate action that serves both self and system. This *Via* reminds us that "Caring is a Passage to the Heart," and on this *Via Positiva* nursing leaders give mindful attention to what has heart.[4]

Via Creativa

Once we have honored the heartfelt journey of the *Via Negativa,* crossed into and learned to dwell in grace and gratitude with the *Via Positiva* of our existence and purpose; once we have begun to more clearly, more consciously assume our voice, our role, and our responsibility for caring and healing for self and system, then we are liberated into new horizons of fresh thinking. On this path of *Via Creativa* we plumb new, deeper dimensions of self and our unique gifts and talents that we can offer as compassionate service on behalf of others. From this *Via Creativa* creative energy and timeless, lasting solutions to our problems become more available, more accessible, more possible, for self and others. From this direction we can creatively return to, articulate, and recreate a larger vision of nursing and health care. From this path the timeless values of caring and the compassionate healing health services manifest more openly, more publicly, as part of our leadership and responsibility for survival of the profession as well as the survival of humane systems of health care.

This *Via* is the Way of the Visionary.[2] When nursing leaders reach this path, they are informed and fortified by nursing ancestors and voices across time that strengthen their vision and purpose, their mindful awareness, attention, and action that flows from the heart of nursing. When on this path, the nursing leader is more able to name that which obstructs and detours basic and humane caring-healing practices for ourselves, our systems, and our public. From this *Via of Leader as Visionary* nurse administrators are empowered from within, more able to tell the truth without blame or judgment.[2] On this *Via of Vision of the Visionary Leader* one is allowed to care enough to make explicit the purpose and deeper meaning that connects and unites the whole value system, reminding self and others why nursing exists, why hospitals exist, why health care systems exist, why caring must be sustained beyond conventional institutional mindsets, and why we seek to move toward a healthful, caring society to better humankind.

Via Transformativa

Finally, in taking this journey of the fourfold path, we enter *Via Transformativa.* On this mature path we have come the full circle of the four sacred directions:

❈ North—*Via Negativa* (the dark—the spiritual warrior)

❈ East—*Via Positiva* (the light—the healer)

❈ West—*Via Creativa* (the water, flow—the visionary)

- South—*Via Transformativa* (the fire—the empowered teacher-leader)

Like an alchemy process, the leader emerges reflective, cleansed, mindful, light-filled, and thus capable of birthing new beings, new possibilities. On the *Via Transformativa* we have co-mingling of leaders and followers, each leading by following his or her own inner call and transformation. Here, having come through the test of fire, often literally as well as figuratively, we are repatterned with new energy to emerge through the alchemy of fire to become the transformative leader, the spirit-filled teacher. From this *Via Transformativa* visionaries, teachers, and healers for systems emerge, leading from the inside out. This form of leadership passes the test of time and position; this transformative leader is able to stand in place, to hold sacred space for caring-healing at all levels while letting go of outcomes,[2] open to outcomes that may never be predicted nor controlled from conventional views of leadership.

Thus, through the fourfold path toward caring and healing, nurse administrators lead, follow, and co-create new forms, orders, and patterns of leadership. By the fourfold path, new levels of consciousness and awareness are more fully actualized, resulting in transformation of self and system.

Taking the fourfold path of leadership allows the growth and integration of the personal and professional journey. From this leading from the inner voice, nursing leaders emerge as spiritual warriors, leaders who are grounded in their own sense of being and becoming, their own *power* with others; connected with and guided by that which is greater than self or system. In this form of deep leadership, the true leader is in balance with the deeper dimensions of life itself. This is the kind of leader who has been on the spiritual journey toward caring and healing in his or her own life.

It is this kind of leader and leadership path by which true transformation occurs. This transformed leader is a visionary, a value-guided navigator toward wholeness and hope. A transformed leader is one who leads from caring, yet follows one's own journey on the fourfold path, honoring the four sacred directions of the universe and the lessons that each direction brings.

How Does One Lead Via the Fourfold Path of Caring and Healing?

To lead *via the fourfold path of caring and healing* is to hear the inner call as to how to translate one's own unique talents and gifts into compassionate service.

To lead *via the fourfold path of caring and healing* is to paradoxically manifest one's full self while simultaneously transcending ego self; to open to connections, visions of the whole, that are greater than any one person but unite all.

To lead *via the fourfold path of caring and healing* is to lead from spirit-filled mindfulness and awareness; to lead by listening to others; to listen to the spirit of what is not said, as much as to what is said; to listen to the sound between the drum beats, detecting the emerging order arising from the comers of the chaos.

To lead *via the fourfold path of caring and healing* is to continuously learn to learn about the sacred circle of life's journey, to awaken to deeper self and human nature, to learn to tap into and affirm the higher, deeper aspects of self and others that embrace and celebrate the diversity of human talents and experiences.

To lead *via the fourfold path of caring and healing* is to learn to pause, to center, to be still, to be authentically present in the midst of hectic paces and demands; to learn to experience a "caring moment" that transcends time and space and allows one to touch and connect spirit to spirit, releasing new energy, new possibilities of what might be, into a given moment.[3]

To lead *via the fourfold path of caring and healing* is to enable self and others; to experiment; to celebrate failures as well as successes, realizing that our failures are our lessons and blessings that transform into new successes; such a consciousness allows the wounds that hurt us to be the wounds that heal us, strengthen us.

To lead *via the fourfold path of caring and healing* is to learn to wait; to dwell in the void, the abyss, and await and co-participate in the order that is emerging out of the chaos; that means attending and being alert to that which wants to emerge as a new path for self and system and society alike. It is often only in waiting that *Via Transformativa* can occur as we pause, on the fourfold journey, on the precipice, in the middle of our sentences, in the middle of our steps, on the sacred walk on the labyrinth of life.

Finally, transformed, nursing leaders reclaim their true vocation, in the full sense of the meaning of the word *vocation;* that is, rooted in the Latin for voice.[5] Transformed nursing leaders at this crossroads in history are giving voice to their mission and vision of caring and healing. Transformed nursing leaders who walk the *fourfold Via* represent hope and order, the other way, for "leadership and the new science,"[6] in the midst of medicalized, industrialized, economized, clinical, and robotic models that are outdated as approaches to human health.

Perhaps it is from the *fourfold Via of caring and healing,* grounded in the spiritual journey of life itself, that leaders are both awaiting and shaping a new world of hope, a new path for new leaders and followers, for new systems, for a renewed health, for all.

In conclusion, as we move forward in this new century of nursing leadership and observe the 25th anniversary of *Nursing Administration Quarterly,* perhaps the *fourfold via* can serve as a useful path to navigate our way through this turn of history in systems of decline, systems in dire need of transformation that can only come from transformed leaders. This fourfold path of leading, which gives voice and informed vocational action to the inner calling of caring and healing, may be the primary source of nursing's survival in this 21st century.

References

1. Fox, M. (1991). *Creation spirituality.* San Francisco: HarperSanFrancisco.
2. Arrien, A. (1993). *The fourfold way.* San Francisco: HarperSanFrancisco.
3. Watson, J. (1999). *Postmodern nursing and beyond.* Edinburgh, Scotland, and New York: Churchill Livingstone/Harcourt-Brace.
4. Watson, J. Brochure information, University of Colorado School of Nursing, Center for Human Caring, 1988.
5. Palmer, P. (2000). *Let your life speak.* San Francisco: Jossey-Bass.
6. Wheatley, M. (1999). *Leadership and the new science.* (2nd ed.). San Francisco: Berrett-Koehler.

References

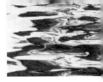

Astin, J. (1991). *Remembrance. A compact disc.* Santa Cruz, CA: Golden Dawn Productions.

Baldwin, C. (1998). *Calling the circle.* New York: Bantam.

Bauman, Z. (1984). *Postmodern ethics.* Oxford, UK: Blackwell.

Benner, P., & Wrubel, J. (1989). *The primacy of caring: Stress and coping in health and illness.* California: Addison Wesley Pub. Co.

Bohm, D. (1980). *Wholeness and the implicate order.* London: Routledge & Kegan Paul.

Brennan, B. (1993). *Light emerging.* New York: Bantam Books.

Chardin, T. (1959). *The phenomenon of man.* New York: Harper & Row.

Critchley, S., & Bernasconi, R. (Eds.), (2002). *The Cambridge companion to Levinas.* Cambridge, UK: Cambridge Press.

Csikszentmihalyi, M. (1990). *Flow the psychology of optimal experience.* New York: HarperCollins.

Day, A. (2003, January). *Keynote.* International Healing Touch Practitioner's (IHTP) Conference, Colorado Springs, CO.

Dossey, L. (1991). *Meaning and medicine.* New York: Bantam.

Dossey, L. (1993). *Healing words.* San Francisco: Harper.

Eagger, S. (2001). Personal communication, International Association of Human Caring conference presentation, University of Stirling, Scotland.

Eliot, T.S. (1944). *Four quartets.* London: Faber & Faber.

Emoto, M. (2002). *Messages from water.* Tokyo, Japan: Hado Publ. Taito-su, (C) I.H.M Co., Ltd.; www.hado.net;book@hado.net.

Eriksson, K. (1997) Caring, spirituality and suffering. In S. Roach (Ed.), *Caring from the heart: The convergence of caring and spirituality* (pp. 68–84). New York: Paulist Press.

Eriksson, K, & Lindstrm U. (1999). A theory of science for caring science. *Hoitotiede, 11*(6), 358–364.

Fawcett, J., Watson, J., Neuman, B., & Hinton-Walker, P. (2001). On theories and evidence. *Journal of Nursing Scholarship, 33*(2), 121–128.

Fiandt, K., Forman, J., Megel, M.E., Pakieser, R.A., & Buirge, S. (2003). Integral nursing: An emerging framework for engaging the evolution of the profession. *Nursing Outlook, 513,* 130–137.

Fincher, S.F. (1991). *Creating mandalas.* Boston: Shambhala.

Fink, M., & MacIntyre, N. (1997). *Introduction to Logstrup's the ethical demand.* Notre Dame (p. xxxiv). Notre Dame, IN: Notre Dame Press.

Fox, M. (1988). *The coming of the cosmic Christ.* New York: Harper & Row.

Gadow, S. (1990). *Beyond dualism and the dialectic of caring and knowing.* Paper presented at Education for Ethical Nursing Practice conference. University of Minnesota: Minneapolis.

Halldorsdottir, S. (1991). Five basic modes of being with another. In D.A. Gaut & M. Leininger (Eds.), *Caring: The compassionate healer.* New York: National League for Nursing.

Hanh, Thich Nhat. (2003). *Creating true peace.* New York: Free Press.

Harman, W. (1991). *A re-examination of the metaphysical foundation of modern science.* Sausalito, CA: Institute of Noetic Sciences.

Harman, W.W. (1990, 1991). Reconciling science and metaphysics. *Noetic Science Review,* 5–10.

Heidegger, M. (1959). *An introduction to metaphysics,* p. 54. (R. Manheim, Trans.). New Haven: Yale University Press.

Heron, J. (1992). *Feeling and personhood: Psychology in another key.* London: Sage.

Hempel, C.G. (1965). *Aspects of Scientific Explanation.* New York, London: Free Press.

Kabat-Zinn, J. (1997). *Gifts of the spirit.* New York: HarperCollins.

Laslett, P. (1956). Introduction to philosophy, politics, and society. In P. Laslett (Series Ed.), & Q. Skinner (Vol. Ed.). (1994). *The return of grand theory,* p. vii. Oxford, UK: Cambridge University.

Levinas, E. (1969). *Totality and infinity* (2000, 14th printing). Pittsburgh, PA: Duquesne University.

Logstrup, K. (1997). *The ethical demand.* Notre Dame, IN: University of Notre Dame Press.

Macrae, J. (1995). Nightingale's philosophy and its significance for modern nursing. *Image: Journal of Nursing Scholarship, 27*(1), 8–10.

Macrae, J. (2001). *Nursing as a spiritual practice.* Philadelphia: FA Davis.

Maslow, A. (1971). *The farther reaches of human nature.* New York: Penguin.

Newman, M. (1992). Prevailing paradigms in nursing. *Nursing Outlook, 40*(1), 10–14.

Newman, M. (1994). Into the 21st century. *Nursing Science Quarterly, 7*(1), 44–46.

Newman, M. (2002). Caring in the human health experience. *International Journal of Human Caring, (6)*2, 8–12.

Newman M.A., Sime A.M., & Corcoran-Perry S.A. (1991). The focus of the discipline of nursing. *Advances in Nursing Science, 14*(1):1–6.

Nortvedt, P. (2000). Clinical sensitivity: The inseparability of ethical perceptiveness and clinical knowledge. *Scholarly Inquiry for Nursing Practice: An International Journal, 14*(3), 1–19.

Nortvedt, P. (2001). Needs, closeness and responsibilities: An investigation into rival moral considerations of nursing care. *Nursing Philosophy, 2*(2), 1–10.

Palmer, P. (1987). Community, conflict and ways of knowing. *Magazine of Higher Learning, 19,* 20–25.

Pearsall, P. (1998). *The heart's code.* New York: Broadway Books/Random House.

Quinn, J., Smith, M., Ritenbaugh, C., Swanson, K., & Watson, J. (2003). Research guidelines for assessing the impact of the healing relationship in clinical nursing. (Reprinted from *Alternative Therapies, 9*[3], A65–A79)

Quinn, J.F. (1992). Holding sacred space: The nurse as healing environment. *Holistic Nursing Practice, 6*(4), 26–35.

Reason, P. (1988). *Human inquiry in action.* London: Sage.

Reason, P. (1993). Reflections on sacred experience and sacred science. *Journal of Management Inquiry 2*(3), 273–283.

Reed, P., Shearer, N., & Nicoll (Eds.), (2003). Perspectives on nursing theory. (4th ed.). New York: Williams and Wilkins.

Roach, S. (1987). *The human act of caring.* The Canadian Hospital Association, Ottawa, Canada.

Rogers, M.E. (1970). *An introduction to theoretical basis of nursing.* Philadelphia: FA Davis.

Rogers M.E. (1992). Nursing science and the space age. *Nursing Science Quarterly, 5,* 27–34.

Rogers, M.E. (1994). The science of unitary human beings. *Nursing Science Quarterly, 2,* 33–35.

Ruiz, D.M. (1999). *The mastery of love. A Toltec wisdom book.* San Rafael, CA: Amber-Allen.

Rumi, J. (2001a). *Hidden music.* M. Mafi, & A. Kolin (Trans.). London: Thorsons/Harper-Collins.

Rumi, J. (2001b). *The glance: Rumi's songs of soul meeting,* p. 12. C. Barks (Trans.). New York: Penguin Compass.

Skinner, Q. (Ed). (1985/reprinted 1994). *The return of grand theory in the human sciences,* p. 10. Cambridge, UK: Cambridge University.

Smith, M. (1994). Arriving at a philosophy of nursing. Discovering? Constructing? Evolving? In J. Kikucki, & H. Simmons (Eds.), *Developing a philosophy of nursing,* pp. 43–60.Thousand Oaks, CA: Sage.

Smith, M. (1999). Caring and the science of unitary human beings. *Advances in Nursing Science, 21*(4), 14–28

Solomon, R.C., & Higgins, K.M. (1997). *A passion for wisdom. A brief history of philosophy.* Oxford, UK: Oxford University.

Swanson, K. (1990). Providing care in the NICU: Sometimes an act of love. *Advances in Nursing Science, 13*(1), 60–73.

Swanson, K. (1991). Empirical development of a middle-range theory of caring. *Nursing Research, 40*(3), 161–166.

Swanson, K. (1999). What is known about caring in nursing research: A literary meta-analysis. In A.S. Hinshaw, S. Feetham, & J. Shaver (Eds.), *Handbook of clinical nursing research,* pp. 31–60. Thousand Oaks, CA: Sage.

Swimme, B. (1996). *The hidden heart of the cosmos,* p. x. Maryknoll, NY: Orbis Books.

Taylor, R. (1974). *Metaphysics* (2nd ed.). Englewood Cliffs, NJ: Prentice-Hall.

Tolle, E. (1999). *The power of now.* Novato, CA: New World Library.

Tolle, E. (2003). *Stillness speaks.* Novato, CA: New World Library.

Vaughn, F. (1995). *Shadows of the sacred.* Wheaton, IL: Quest Books.

Waldman, A. (2001) *Vow to poetry.* Minneapolis: Coffee House Press.

Watson, J. (1985). *Nursing: The philosophy and science of caring.* Boulder, CO: Colorado Associated University Press.

Watson, J. (1988, 1999). *Nursing: Human science and human care.* New York: National League for Nursing. (Reprinted Sudbury, Mass: Jones & Bartlett.)

Watson, J. (1995). Nursing's caring-healing paradigm as exemplar for alternative medicine? *Journal of Alternative Therapies in Health and Medicine, 1*(3), 64–69.

Watson J. (1999a). *Nursing: Human Science and Human Caring. A Theory of Nursing.* Sudbury, Mass: Jones & Bartlett.

Watson J. (1999b). *Postmodern nursing and beyond.* Edinburgh, Scotland: Churchill Livingstone/Harcourt-Brace.

Watson, J. (2000). Leading via caring-healing: The fourfold way toward transformative leadership. *Nursing Administration Quarterly, 25*(1): 1–6.

Watson, J. (2002). *Assessing and measuring caring in nursing and health science,* pp. 13–14. New York: Springer.

Watson, J. (2002). Intentionality and caring-healing consciousness: A practice of transpersonal nursing. *Journal of Holistic Nursing Practice, 16*(4):12–19.

Watson, J. (2002). Metaphysics of virtual caring communities. *International Journal of Human Caring, 6*(1), 41–45.

Watson, J. (2003) Love and caring: Ethics of face and hand. *Nursing Administration Quarterly, 27*(3):197–202.

Watson, J., & Smith, M. (2002). Caring science and the science of unitary human beings: A trans-theoretical discourse for nursing knowledge development. *Journal of Advanced Nursing, 37*(5), 452–461.

Weber, R. (1986). *Dialogues with scientists and sages: The search for unity.* London: Routledge & Kegan Paul.

Whitehead, A.N. (1925). *Science and the modern world.* New York: Free Press

Wilber, K. (1982). *The holographic paradigm.* Boston: Shambhala.

Wilber, K. (1998) *The essential Ken Wilber.* Boston: Shambhala.

Wilber, K. (2001).
   http://wilber.shambhala.com/html/misc/haberman/index.cfm/xid,5837/yid,5049275
Wilber, K., & Walsh, R. (2000). An integral approach to consciousness research. In *Investigating phenomenal consciousness: New methodologies and maps*. Philadelphia: John Benjamins.
Williamson, M. (1992). *Return to love*. New York: Harper Perennial.
Zukav, G. (1990). *The seat of the soul*. New York: Fireside, Simon & Shuster.